HIV Infected by Her Cheating Pastor Husband

A WIFE'S COURAGEOUS TRUE STORY OF BETRAYAL, SURVIVAL AND FORGIVENESS

by
Darlene King

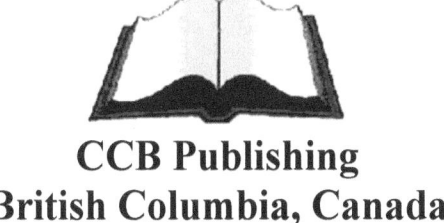

CCB Publishing
British Columbia, Canada

HIV Infected by Her Cheating Pastor Husband:
A Wife's Courageous True Story of
Betrayal, Survival and Forgiveness

Copyright ©2012 by Darlene King
ISBN-13   978-1-927360-86-6
First Edition

Library and Archives Canada Cataloguing in Publication
King, Darlene, 1959-
HIV infected by her cheating pastor husband : a wife's courageous true story of betrayal, survival and forgiveness / by Darlene King – 1st ed.
ISBN 978-1-927360-86-6
Also available in electronic format.
Additional cataloguing data available from Library and Archives Canada

Scriptures taken from *The Holy Bible, King James Version*.
New York: Oxford Edition: 1769; *King James Bible Online*, 2008.
http://www.kingjamesbibleonline.org/ Used by permission.
All rights reserved worldwide.

Scriptures taken from *The Holy Bible, King James Version Reference Bible*, Copyright © 1994 by The Zondervan Corporation. Published by Zondervan, Grand Rapids, Michigan 49530, U. S. A. Used by permission of Zondervan. All rights reserved worldwide http://www.zondervan.com The "NIV" and "New International Version" are trademarks registered in the United States Patent and Trademark Office by Biblica, Inc.™

Extreme care has been taken to ensure that all information presented in this book is accurate and up to date at the time of publishing. Neither the author nor the publisher can be held responsible for any errors or omissions. Additionally, neither is any liability assumed for damages resulting from the use of the information contained herein.

All rights reserved. No part of this publication may be reproduced, stored in a retrieval system or transmitted in any form or by any means, electronic, mechanical, photocopying, recording or otherwise without the express written permission of the publisher. Printed in the United States of America, the United Kingdom and Australia.

Publisher: CCB Publishing
               British Columbia, Canada
               www.ccbpublishing.com

*This book is dedicated to my parents and children.
I have been blessed with the most supportive
Parents anyone could ever ask for.
Unconditional love poured from them daily.
In spite of all my shortcomings,
they've encouraged and lifted my spirits.
Mom I miss you more than words can express.
The legacy of Love you left continues to flow.
Dad, you truly are the best dad in the world,
and I thank God for you daily
To my girls,
Who could ask for more patient and supportive daughters?
My decisions have caused you undue hardship, but
through it all you have trusted God, and allowed
Him to develop you into the beautiful ladies you
have become. Continue to hold on to
God's unchanging hand.*

Acknowledgements

I would like to acknowledge
my Pastor and his beautiful Wife
and all the members of our congregation.
Your encouragement and support towards
our family has been a true blessing.

I would also like to acknowledge
Mary Hale and Bonnie Kaye.
I Thank God for the young man who
lead me to the both of you.
I am forever grateful for
your support and encouragement.

To the most supportive sisters in the world,
Thank You.

To my niece Nikki, Thank You for coming to my
bedside every time I am sick.

To my niece Jenny, Thank You for all your care in
taking the cover photos.

To All of You Many Thanks
and May God Continually Bless You

Contents

My Voice of Healing 1
Chapter 1   An Unplanned Downfall 5
Chapter 2   Days Spent in a Haze 11
Chapter 3   Suffering in Silence 16
Chapter 4   Utter Blindness 23
Chapter 5   Sickness That Refuses to Let Go 27
Chapter 6   I'm in Church, Let's Talk 35
Chapter 7   How Did I End Up with the Title? 63
Chapter 8   Pain Like You Wouldn't Believe 83
Chapter 9   Wake Up! You're Suffering from
            Depression 87
Chapter 10 Who Am I Really? 99
Chapter 11 One of Those Days 108
Chapter 12 No I Didn't End Up in Another Crazy
            Emergency Room 110
Chapter 13 Why Write? 116
Chapter 14 My Year of Jubilee 119
Chapter 15 A Sermon Worth Sharing 131
Chapter 16 Why Are There So Many Questions
            After Death? 147
Chapter 17 Lessons Learned As We Head for
            the Inevitable 155
Chapter 18 There Will Be Pain and Joy 164
About the Author 172

My Voice of Healing

(Isaiah 53:5 kjv)
*"But he was wounded for our transgressions,
he was bruised for our iniquities:
the chastisement of our peace was upon him;
and with his stripes we are healed."*

I have awoken this morning with a rash on my face. You would not believe the fear that settles in with every sore, rash, and cut. My first thought is, is this going to heal? Will it get worse? Where did it come from? I'm looking in the mirror telling myself all the things I have been taught from valiant women of God. "Beauty is in the eye of the beholder." "It doesn't matter what my face looks like, it's what's in my heart." I am telling myself that I can never be so vain as to not go out and serve God, regardless of what my face looks like. This is why I am getting dressed to go to church. But the reality is it brings back the horror of all the diseases I have contracted in this relationship which will one day have me serve as the First Lady of our church with my husband serving as the Pastor. With each new sore or sickness, your thoughts immediately go to death. Everyone knows that someday they will die, but people who suffer with HIV and AIDS know that the reality of a compromised immune system could spell instant deterioration if our weakened defenses are no longer able to fight.

I always feared these rashes all over my face. I remember he would get them all the time. I would plead with him to go to the doctors. But the response was, "It's only an allergic reaction to something I have eaten."

There were so many lies. Sometimes I wondered was anything the truth? Will I ever know what the rashes truly were? Can I contract it? What's next? But today, I am hit with a powerful sense that this could have been my spiritual death and not the death from this disease. God will take care of me as I die from the ravages of this disease. But what if I had not freed myself from the wickedness and evil in which I was surrounded? The thought that I could have died while my soul was gripped in utter agony and sadness was painful. The thought of sitting another Sunday in worship to an all mighty God as the dutiful First Lady while inside I am in misery is overwhelming. In the absence of love and good the only thing left that could exist for me is hate and evil. Who in their right mind would choose to worship in such a state? No thank you. I'm good. At least now anyway. Anyone who chooses can remain in that space all by herself. As for me and my house we're out.

In front of me stands my husband--the Pastor--whom I haven't seen since he received his paycheck on Friday. I don't know why this particular Sunday came flooding back to my mind today as I look in the mirror at this rash, but I smile because I was set free, September 5, 2003, and counting. You'll find that these days I love counting. With each day that I can add, I praise God that my body is no longer being defiled through spirits of unknown origin that may enter every time I lay down with my spouse. Worship is all that I have. I will never allow anyone or anything to interfere with my worship.

Worship is what God requires. How many other First Ladies, Deaconesses, Pastors, Deacons, women and men of God dread this coming Sunday because they know that they have to put on their happy face and dutifully serve? How many others still suffer in silence? Whose actions right at this moment as I write is about to bring disease and suffering and tear down the structure of their families for generations to come out of such a trivial act of lustful disobedience to a

Faithful God? So I had to write because someone may be saved. Someone may be delivered. Someone may be set Free.

"For he whom the Son set's Free, is truly Free indeed." (John 8:36 kjv) God requires Faithfulness. God requires Obedience. *"Be not deceived; God is not mocked: for whatsoever a man soweth, that shall he also reap." (Galatians 6:7 kjv)*

Chapter 1

An Unplanned Downfall

(John 1:1-2 kjv) "In the beginning was the Word, and the Word was with God, and the Word was God. 2He was with God in the beginning."

I'm trying to think of when the deterioration began. When did my life begin to unravel? Then I think just like man's deterioration began in the Garden of Eden when Adam sinned against God, my deterioration began with sexual sins against God.

Whoever thinks of sex as one of the most powerful weapons Satan has to use against mankind? But at age 52, I have the hindsight to see that as for me, this sin against God truly was the beginning of everything falling apart. There is a reason that God requires consummation between husband and wife only. Spirits can only be transferred from one individual to another by two ways. One is laying on of hands.

(I Timothy 5:22 kjv) "Lay hands suddenly on no man, neither be partaker of other men's sins: keep thyself pure."

The other way spirits can be transferred is sex.

(Genesis 2:24 kjv) "Therefore shall a man leave his father and his mother, and shall cleave unto his wife: and they shall be one flesh."

Here the scripture tells us that the two shall become one. Spirits are transferred between the two individuals at the time of consummation. The two are therefore intertwined and have now become one spirit.

Now picture this: If a woman is promiscuous, over time she has had sex with 10 to 20 different folks. And a man also had sex with 10 to 20 different folks. And all those 10 to 20 different individuals also had sex with 10 to 20 different people. Guess how many spirits we have now become one with? Now I'm sure there are a whole lot of spirits, which have now become apart of me, that I did not bargain for when I decided to have sex. Nor do I want them to become a part of my future.

Just imagine that at the moment you lay down with an individual, you look up and see approximately 440 different faces of all the spirits you are about to become intertwined with just by sleeping with this one individual. And in each face you are able to read all kinds of personalities. You see jealousy, lying, cheating, hatred, malice, demons, drunks, crack addicts, cocaine addicts, marijuana addicts, and thieves.

You would jump up out of that bed so fast that you would probably run out of the house naked, running so fast, the people on the street would not even be able to tell you were naked. You would be like a streak that just flew by. Zoooom… But unfortunately, hindsight is the only way you will be able to see what you are really allowing to enter this temple of God that he has kindly asked us to *"present your bodies a living sacrifice, holy, acceptable unto God, which is your reasonable service." (Romans 12:1 kjv)*

There are a whole lot of folks running around inside of us. Picture a husband or wife goes out to cheat on his or her spouse. The individual he or she sleeps with has had sex with hundreds of people. The individual they sleep with is at that moment struggling with alcohol addiction, crack addiction, or cocaine addiction. Or maybe he or she sleeps with someone who has HIV, gonorrhea, syphilis, or some other sexually transmitted disease. Now you went out there just to sneak off for one night of sex. You come home and sleep with your spouse. Now both of you have a disease, possibly one you cannot cure.

One may begin an addiction because you took the

crack pipe from another party before you had sex, just to get the edge off so you could go through with this act. Now you have a crack addiction because after that first hit, you just had to have another.

Do you see the powerful tool sex becomes? It becomes a weapon in which we have given Satan the power to use against us. And I can tell you from experience, there is no sex in the world worth losing your health, spouse, home, car, marriage, children, job, finances, family, or friends over. But that's exactly what we let one little sex act do--bring all kinds of suffering into our homes. All it takes is having sex once with the wrong individual to tear down your entire family. Is it worth it? NO! But we know that's not really happening all over this world, right? Keep it real. I'm not in this boat all by myself. So to the folks who are in my boat, it's okay. The Captain of all Captains is about to save us.

(1 John 1:9 kjv) "If we confess our sins, He is faithful and just to forgive us our sins, and to cleanse us from all unrighteousness."

Sex then becomes this powerful tool because it has been the source of the destruction of so many families for so many years. I am sure if you ask many of the people who are going through divorce or a break-up what happened, sex or money will be at the root of many of the issues. And men, please listen to me. There is a tradition out there to take your sons when they turn 13 or over to have sex with a prostitute. I wouldn't do that if I were you. The day and age of doing that is dead. You can do it if you want to. I pray the condom doesn't break because that little act of what you think is making him into a man unfortunately may be coming back to haunt you. Here's God's description of a real man. And if all parents are honest with themselves, this is how they want the man they raise to be described.

(Psalm 1:1-2 kjv) "Blessed is the man that walketh not in the counsel of the ungodly, nor standeth in the way of sinners, nor sitteth in the seat of the scornful.

But his delight is in the law of the LORD; and in his law doth he meditate day and night."

Some people say that the love and relationships that we see on the big screen don't exist. But I feel that any type of love you desire exists in the form in which you are willing to give. Two individuals have the power to touch and agree on the bond and relationship they are willing to commit their lives to. Both have the power within themselves to love one another exactly with the type of love they desire. And if they are on the same page, in total commitment to give of themselves, and their desires of what they want to achieve are in agreement, a love like never before will exist. God can give each of you a pure love that you couldn't even begin to imagine existed. Eyes have not seen, nor ears heard, what God can do when we totally trust him with everything, even how to love my spouse.

Chapter 2

Days Spent in a Haze

There was a reason that I shared those specific spirits that are transferred through sex. I named those specific sins against God only because there was a time in which each became my name. From experience, I know its ravages of self destruction. I have come to know personally the depths of darkness some will sink to in order to get their next high. Oh, the stories of my stupidity. I believe the worst position to be in when you're a drug addict is to not know where the places are to buy drugs. You are then at the mercy of all the other people around you who get high, to buy their drugs for them every time you want to buy drugs. For years since I was a teenager, I supported the habits of at least 10 different individuals. That does not include the countless others who have gotten high at my expense.

It breaks my heart to sometimes count the thousands of dollars spent over so many years. But then the worst part was constantly being gagged. I would pay for 4 or 5 bags of cocaine, and they come back with bags of the stuff you cut the drugs with claiming the drug dealer scammed them. You know what my stupidity would have me do next. Give them more money for another 4 or 5 bags, just for them to come back and say the same thing.

You know it was years later when I was sober that I realized I put my money in the hands of individuals who were just as addicted as me and expected them to come back and deliver me drugs. But there is a part of me that is so glad for all the scams. When God was ready for me to come out for good, I got so fed up with the last scam of my drug life that I never smoked nor snorted again. Another episode that helped deliver me from crack was a night that I was smoking and began to shake. I was so scared I thought I would die. In that instant God gave me a moment of clarity. As clear as day I heard, what if I die and go to hell right in the middle of smoking this crack? I was literally scared straight. Talk about your eye opener. But my experience has been that crack cocaine was the most addictive drug I have ever taken.

From the day I first smoked crack, I could not get enough. It takes you over completely. You go to sleep thinking about it; you wake up thinking about it. Just by someone flicking a match, you think of smoking. But the craziest thing was, I could work all day not smoking, but that was the first thing I had to have the moment I got off of work. I have never smoked crack while I was working. So if I can control this during the day, why can't I control it during the evening? When you smoke crack it goes to your brain instantly. The first thing I noticed was my hearing became really sharp, and I could hear everything. Every step, every movement, every sound would make me jump. I would start locking doors and closing windows. Complete paranoia would take over. This was no fun at all, but I couldn't stop.

It's sad for me to admit this, but the only thing I liked about crack was the weight loss. Even today, needing to lose a lot of weight, I always think about crack. Not thinking that I want it, but why can't they figure out exactly what it is in crack that makes you lose weight and then put this in a pill so I can lose weight, without getting high and spending thousands of dollars?

I thank God the desire is completely gone. The craziest scams came from my days of smoking crack. "I have a hole in my pocket, so they must have fallen out of my pocket." "I gave him the money, and he told me to wait, but he never came back." "This is all that came in the bottle. It was dark, and I didn't see it until I got in the light." "I gave him a twenty, and he said it was only a five." "I must have lost the money." After you have sat an entire night waiting for someone to come back with the drugs, you finally catch up with them the next day and hear, "I was jumped, and someone took the money, so I just went home." And guess what? You then give them some more money to go and buy drugs that you still may never see. I was scammed so much, I can not even remember all the different crazy stories I was told during those drug induced years.

I was introduced to cocaine on my 21st birthday. That was supposed to be my birthday present. If someone is offering you cocaine as a present, run as fast as you can.

That's not a present; they are looking for a financial backer. They are going down, and if they can get you hooked, they'll have another person to finance their habit. So don't do it. And just in case you end up as stupid as I was, make sure you know some prayer warriors. Much prayer is the only thing that can bring you out. My situation was that nothing but Jesus Christ himself could get me off drugs. Trust me on this one because I know what I am talking about. I came off that stuff only by the grace of God. I could have gone to all the rehabs I wanted. But until I turned my life over completely to God, nothing worked. That's my own personal experience. I am not knocking rehabilitation facilities. Some people really need these facilities and they have done individuals a lot of good. Some people cannot come off of drugs without rehabilitation. Turn to what works for you. But please get help.

God alone pulled me out. I know there are some that will still have a need to try this for themselves. So, I stand in the ready, to pray. Trust me, you're going to need prayer if you start that mess. I know some folks who have a relationship with God who are in constant prayer, and they will be able to get a prayer through on your behalf. So, if by some chance you are able to get your brain working for a second, find a way to call some prayer warriors. And if you can't, drop on your knees at start praying for yourself.

(James 5:16 kjv) "Confess your faults one to another, and pray one for another that ye may be healed. The effectual fervent prayer of a righteous man avails much."

Chapter 3

Suffering in Silence

As I began to write this week, I thought of a prominent First Lady of one of our country's governors. She stated on Oprah that she called a former First Lady of the United States because she was the first person she thought of who could relate to her suffering. I do not presume to even begin to compare myself to these beautiful strong women who had to endure public humiliation. But I was talking to the TV, as I often do, screaming, "You are not alone! There are many who have suffered your fate, and no one will ever come to know their names. Not just First Ladies, but men and women all over this world. They may not have a title, but suffering knows no title."

You hear so often of women being abused and taken advantage of, but there are many men who also suffered our same fate. Our names are known only by our congregations, communities, families, children, friends, and co-workers. The people who are most important in our lives are the ones we worry about, especially when they have found out what we are going through. And this group for me seems like the world. We always say it doesn't matter what others think, but in reality it does. It hurts because in most cases, when you have suffered public humiliation, all those around you whom you love the most have also been hurt.

Several things happened for me to finally wake up and free myself from being surrounded by wickedness. I was in church one Sunday, in my place in the front pew. I always sit up front, so I usually don't see what's going on behind me. Only God knows what made me turn around this particular day. The moment that I turned around, I saw a look on my daughter's face that sent chills through my body. She had a look of utter disgust as her step-father was preaching. She looked so sad, miserable and lonely. I instantly wanted to cry. At that moment I realized that my silent suffering had transferred to my children. Feelings that I thought were only affecting me had begun to affect my household. I did not share with the children all my suspicions and doubts. But clearly, they also have a sense that something is not right.

I decided at that moment that no one should be this miserable in Worship Service. We are there to glorify

God. God can't be glorified if our hearts are in such a terrible state. I stopped going to Sunday worship, and I would no longer send my children.

My daughter had good reason for looking the way she did. First of all, children are not stupid. You may think you are discussing your family problems in the confines of your bedroom, trying to shield your children from what's really going on. But believe me, actions speak louder than words. You say one thing to them, but treat them in a totally different way. You think they don't know what you really feel? They know you haven't been home all week and that their mother has no clue where you are. Our son is calling your cell phone for days, and you never return the call. Then you show up early Sunday morning demanding everyone get up to go to church, and we are supposed to be happy and smiling about this situation. I don't think so.

Another eye opener was being told, "I married beneath me." It was unbelievable for me to hear these words from someone who at this point is on crack, cocaine, marijuana, and sleeping with every prostitute he can afford. Someone who drops in Sunday morning to preach God's word, then leaves for days. This individual has enough nerve to say to me, "I married beneath me." I felt at that moment I had spent most of my life loving someone who sounds as if they don't even like me let alone love me. I am feeling like he despises me and that he despises women. My husband, who will soon not even attend his mother's home going service, says, "I married beneath me." I was in total disbelief.

At first I felt like I had given so much to someone who did not deserve it. But this was all for a purpose. This was all in God's plan. I was supposed to receive this wake up call. I have learned every lesson I was meant to learn. Without a doubt this season came to an end and it was time to leave. It came to an end in God's time. Every lesson learned is now to be used to help others suffering the same distress. I will be able to testify, witness and encourage others who feel they have spent their lives unloved. We need to be reminded that God was always with us. In spite of what it looked and felt like, God never left us nor forsaken us. We were always loved unconditionally.

Now prior to this point, I didn't even know all of this was going on, but I knew something is going on. He's not at work, he's not at home, and something is not right. With an eye opening calm, and a resolute smile, I say, "No, I married beneath me." I smiled because at that moment I realized he knew he never deserved my dedication and commitment to this marriage. It had never crossed my mind to think or even say another human being is beneath me. One thing that keeps me focused was the realization, that I was, and would always be a sinner, saved by Gods' grace.

If it were not for the grace of God, I would be dead. I appreciate what God had done for me. I had sunk to the depths of self destruction. It was only God who picked me up from darkness and despair and saved me. What could ever make me think that I am in a position to degrade another individual? The thought that a person could look down on an individual and even let the words "beneath me" roll off their lips made me angry. But I am thankful for those words. Years of clarity came into being with the utterance of those four words. For at that moment I could clearly see what was behind years of infidelity.

Our Love was not mutual. Disdain now lies where love may have lain at some point in time. I saw what lied in the depths of his heart. And I knew beyond a shadow of a doubt that this was the end. I know you're probably thinking it should have ended a long time ago. But, every season runs its course. And the end came when it was time. Lord, keep me humble, lest I fall flat on my face.

I was just thinking of that story from the Book of Daniel, Chapter 4, when God had to reduce Nebuchadnezzar down to a stump because of his pride. God please don't let me get so high and mighty that you have to knock me down to a stump to the point where I have to eat grass like the cattle. I thank you Jesus for hanging out with the least of us.

(Matthew 25:40 kjv) "And the King shall answer and say unto them, Verily I say unto you, Inasmuch as ye have done it unto one of the least of these my brethren, ye have done it unto me."

You don't need a title to confirm that you are first. You are first in the eyes of God. I can tell you that you are first because you were uniquely created for God's pleasure. He has an individual plan for each of us, and every one of us is special in his eyes. *"There is Joy in heaven over just one, that turns back to God." (Luke 15:7 kjv)*

This is not to say that we live a life for just self-- quite the opposite. This is to acknowledge that when life tears us down and feelings of hopelessness begin to set in, we must find the strength to begin to look at ourselves as God looks at us.

*(Ephesians 1:4-6 kjv) "For he chose us in him before the creation of the world, to be holy and blameless in his sight. In love he predestined us to be adopted as his sons through Jesus Christ, in accordance with his pleasure and will to the praise of his glorious grace, which he has freely given us in the **One** he loves."*

I am created for his pleasure. That statement alone is enough for us to get happy and rejoice. If all that I am hearing in the issues that I face in life is that I am nothing. I am worthless. Then move away from the negative and move toward the prize.

(Isaiah 49:13 kjv) "Shout for joy, O heavens; rejoice, O earth; burst into song, O mountains! For the Lord comforts his people and will have compassion on his afflicted ones."

Chapter 4

<u>Utter Blindness</u>

It's funny when I think back to this incident how my eyes were opened. We were dropping off the friend of our youngest son, whom he played basketball with on the weekends. The moment his mom reached the car, I looked into her eyes. The look of affection and longing I saw on her face was unmistakable. Then I looked into my husband's eyes, and I knew instantly he was sleeping with her. I couldn't say a word because all the children were in the car. In my head I am screaming! He has me babysitting while he is sleeping with her! I could not get him alone fast enough. I confronted him and he denied it. He insisted he was not sleeping with her. He must have told her because she had the nerve to call and inform me that they were going to be together. I said, "Did he tell you he had HIV?" I could tell by the silence he had not. She called me several days later to tell me that I lied. He told her I lied just to keep them apart. I told her she could have him, but just make sure you get tested in six months, and then you'll know who is lying. Now I know he wasn't using a condom because this fiasco--like many that had come and would come soon again--resulted in him telling me she might be pregnant.

I confronted him as to how he could be having sex with this woman and not tell her he was HIV positive? The response and I quote was, "She used to be a prostitute, so she probably already has it." I'm screaming, you're a minister why are you doing this? This young lady's son played basketball with my youngest son. So he would spend the weekends with us when they had a game. I was the babysitter for her son, while my husband spent the weekends with her. Now I know you are thinking--she stayed with that fool even after that? I have no answer, but in my case love was blind, deaf, dumb, stupid, and reality had left the building.

This is why I am sitting here at this computer; some man or woman might still have a chance. Boy, how many times had I kicked myself over that one? Man, I was almost out. I left again, but he convinced me to come back. I could have just said, "Okay, you win." But there was more humiliation to come. For the life of me, I just can't comprehend how anyone could have sex with another person and not tell her they have this disease. The thought that there are many people infecting others without a thought or care for the life of that individual escapes me. I wish I could say, "Please do unto others as you would have done unto yourself." Would it be okay for someone to purposely infect your grandmother? Would it be okay for someone to purposely infect your son or daughter? Would it be okay to infect someone's mother or father?" Of course it would not be okay! Everyone on this planet is special to someone. It you don't care about them, then leave them to those who care. Place yourself in someone's shoes, and imagine what you have done, coming back on your family. Not a pretty picture I am sure. If we really believe the scripture that we reap what we sow, then could the things we do come back on one of our family members? This gives us something to think about for sure. Lord please place a hedge around my family, and forgive me for all that I have done to others. May their lives be full, rich and blessed by You. Amen.

There needs to be an ad campaign reminding people of the number of years they can go to jail for intentionally infecting someone, without their knowledge. I bet if reminded of the threat of jail, some people wouldn't be so callous in just passing it around, like they are passing someone a mint or a piece of gum. There are people out there with a mentality that someone gave it to me, so I will give it to someone else. This is crazy. Please don't do anything this foolish. I don't care who you are. In this life you reap what you sow. You will have to answer to God one day for everything you have said and done.

(Romans 14:12 kjv) "So then every one of us shall give account of himself to God."

Chapter 5

Sickness That Refuses to Let Go

Being sick with HIV has been the most depressing aspect of my life. There are times that I feel so good, that I forget I have HIV. I can go days of being up and jolly, with no symptoms in sight. A commercial may come on TV talking about HIV, and I say to myself, "I almost forgot I have HIV!" When I am with my church family and friends, I don't even think about it. Then there are days, like today, when reality sets in. At this moment as I write, I am on 19 different medications. Some I take 2 or 3 times a day. And one I take 5 times a day. Right now the feeling of wanting to vomit is so strong it makes my stomach hurt even more just thinking about it. It's a good thing my daughters aren't home. Writing this is making me cry, and I never want them to see me cry. The times I've let them see me cry hurts even more when I see the worry and pain across their faces. When they see me cry, then they start crying. They are so brave. I could use a little of their bravery right now.

I cry a lot when I am by myself. "You're an Evangelist; you're not supposed to cry." Yeah, right. I cry so much it's not even funny. People always say, "You are always so happy; you are always smiling." And that's true I really am very happy even though you can't tell, at this moment, through these tears. But these days I cry even when I am not sad. Ever since I found that scripture from Psalm 56:8 that my tears are in God's bottle, I have no problem crying. I imagine every drop falling into God's bottle. I wrote a song from that scripture.

Wait a minute, I just thought of something funny. It was on a television show when every time someone would say something, they would follow it up saying something like they wrote a song about whatever was the topic. I cannot remember which television show this was on. In any case, it just made me laugh, so now I am laughing and crying at the same time. It's not like the medications I took today are any different than the ones I've been taking for years. So why today am I so sick? I can't count the days like this. I am gripped with diarrhea from the moment I wake up in the morning. I try to eat just so I can take this medicine, but the thought of food makes me sick. I think I am the fattest sick person in the world. Anyone else who has diarrhea every day would probably lose weight; nope, not me. I get all the pleasures of this sickness, without the weight loss.

I am so nauseous that I am dizzy. Just walking to the bathroom is making me short of breath. I can't tell if it's the HIV or the diabetes. But I just checked my sugar levels, and they are okay. The neuropathy is sending pain shooting from behind my knees. The agony from my back and neck pain is not going to allow me to sit at this computer much longer. But I need to get this feeling at this moment down on paper. My eyes are blurry from my tears. How is it possible that a person's eyeballs can hurt? I have such a bad headache. When it hurts this bad, I always think, "Do I have a brain tumor?"

I feel lonely, but as soon as I spoke the word loneliness into my spirit, Jesus spoke, *"I will never leave you nor forsake you."* (Hebrew 13:5 kjv) I keep drinking water because I do not want to get dehydrated. I hate the emergency room. No, let me rephrase that--I dislike the emergency room. Hate is a strong word and a feeling I do not wish to have in my spirit. There have been days just like this, and that's where I ended up at the end of the day. My heart feels like someone is squeezing my chest. I have a heart murmur. And I keep getting these palpitations. I am thinking please don't throw up on this computer; I don't have enough money to buy another one.

I am already trying to figure out today how I am going to pay to get my car fixed. I know I should be calling my family, but for some reason when I am the sickest, I don't want them to know. They would think I'm crazy for sitting there all day with chest pains. My family worries about me so much. They don't think I know, but I do. Just like my children, they watch over me for any signs that I may be getting worse.

I have the best family in the world. I am the youngest girl. And my sisters would give their last breath for me. This is how they make me feel. My sisters are so overprotective of me. If I told them someone treated me unkindly, they would be like, "Who, what, when, where? Tell me right now Di, where are they? What did they say to you?" Especially my one sister--she's too crazy. She would track somebody down for hurting me. She's already going to get me when she finds out all the things that have happened that she will find out about once she reads this book.

I hope other people are blessed with wonderful

families who care so much for them. But I know that there are many who don't have such wonderful support. "Father in the name of Jesus, I pray that you surround all those who are in need with your Love, Care and Kindness. If they are in need of support, please bring, God, more support than they can begin to imagine. In Jesus name I pray. Amen." All you family members out there, show your people some Love. I know I just digressed, but that will happen a lot. Just typing exactly what comes to mind. Anyway, if this is the day God chooses to call me home. It is well with my soul.

Don't get me wrong--I don't want to die. I have two of the most beautiful daughters in the world. I want to be here a long time to see them become all that God has in store for them. And recently all I keep thinking about is grandchildren. By golly I think I am ready for some grandkids. But I want God to allow me to live long enough to see my daughters graduate from college, get a job, get married, and then bring me some grandkids. I know I am asking for a lot. *"But you have not because you ask not." (James 4:2 kjv)*

But when you get this weak this often, how can you not think about death? About a month ago, I had a fever that lasted for over four days. By the fourth day, the chills were so bad it felt like someone was sticking needles all over my body. I did everything I could to try and make myself sweat. I thought if I could just sweat, my body temperature would regulate. In the midst of this, all I could think about was there are people even sicker than I am with HIV and AIDS who have had fevers for months. Can you imagine the pain they are in? Those little four days were nothing compared to the people who aren't even able to stand up. Even then I wouldn't go to the emergency room. By the fourth day, my poor daughter wanted to drag me to the hospital. I refused to go because people in the emergency room can be so cold, cruel, and judgmental. I have gone to the emergency room and had the most compassionate people on the planet take care of me. But many times it is the exact opposite. I recall this one occasion when they placed me in a room and took some blood. They asked me a few questions and then left me there for the next five hours by myself. I am dozing in and out, but I can hear them talking right outside of the room about me as if I don't even exist.

Oxycodin was one of the pain killers on my medication list. I keep my medication list in my purse because this is the first thing they ask for anytime I go to the hospital. And my list is too long to remember all the names and dosages of each prescription. This particular day I did not take the Oxycodin and had not taken it for weeks because my stomach was upset, and I knew it would upset my stomach even more. The doctor and nurse stood outside my room laughing and talking about me as if I wasn't even there, speculating that it was most likely the Oxycodin because I was dozing off. I wanted to scream, I am dozing off, because it's 5:00 a.m. in the morning, and I have been here since 8:00 p.m. the night before. And the first four hours of being here consisted of sitting in a cold lobby, in a cold hard chair, with chills--freezing, wondering if this was going to be the night I die. I am listening to them talk about me and thinking, I could have stayed in my bed for all this.

If I am leaving this earth, let it be in a place where I know I am loved. This is why today that is exactly where I am staying--in my bed. Okay, between this pain shooting across my shoulders and fear of throwing up all over my computer, I have to end this chat. Lord please allow me to live long enough to spoil my future grandchildren. And Lord, please help me to forgive anyone who has ever treated me wrong in the hospital. And Jesus, just in case I end up there tonight, let me be greeted by some really nice people.

(Luke 6:37 kjv) "Judge not, and ye shall not be judged: condemn not, and ye shall not be condemned: forgive, and ye shall be forgiven."

Chapter 6
<u>I'm in Church, Let's Talk</u>

Why do our churches have such a hard time talking about and dealing with HIV and AIDS? I've had some very interesting experiences on this issue. As a person facing death from this disease, I think it is time to talk. No, we are way past time to talk, it is crucial that we talk. The word says train up a child in the way he or she should go. *(Proverbs 22:6)* If we don't teach our children, then the streets will teach them. Unfortunately, then it may be too late.

We are telling children don't have sex. It's a sin against God, and you may get pregnant. Now yes, that is true. But in this day and age there's some more stuff that needs to be added to our birds and the bees talk. These days the birds and the bees are not even safe. What makes you think our children are safe? Birds are dying from West Nile Virus disease. Bees are dying off by colonies, and no one knows why. Our children are contracting this disease because no one is being real with them and in the process, dying off in record numbers.

Tell them the old saying, "You lie down with dogs, you may come up with fleas." Well baby that has drastically changed. You lie down with anybody, and you may come up with AIDS. Don't have sex because it's a sin against God if you are not married, and also, you may get AIDS or other sexually transmitted diseases you will never be able to get rid of. You may get pregnant, and then transmit the disease to your unborn child. You're only a teenager, therefore the likelihood that you will be with this boy for the rest of your life is unlikely. And since you both now have this disease, the rest of both of your lives have just been cut short because you now have AIDS. Not only your life, but the life of all the people you have had sex with, and the lives of all the people he has had sex with, since you both contracted this disease. We do not know if you or your child will live through this disease. But both of you now require going on medications for the rest of your life, how ever long that may be.

Now some might say you don't have to be that dramatic. And I would say they probably don't have AIDS or HIV. Trust me. We don't want our children to suffer the same fate as we have suffered especially if it's a painful fate. The first time I spoke of HIV was at a women's prayer breakfast at my old church. I really felt I was in a room with people who loved me. I needed help and the support of other women. I shared my testimony and then just broke down crying. When I opened my eyes the first thing I noticed is that some of the older women were no longer holding my hands. They had moved away from me. A few of them never really got too close to me. I was being held up by two beautiful women. I thank God for them. They know who they are. I felt like I no longer had to hide behind this disease. From that moment on I found some true friends who have supported me with unconditional love. A couple of them just came to my church to support me on a day that I was scheduled to preach. Thank you from the bottom of my heart. Unfortunately my husband was livid. He was so angry that I told people at church. For years every time we would get in an argument he would bring up the story about me telling the women at church. We could be having a disagreement over dinner and he would bring up me telling the women. I think I shrunk an area of people he could prey on.

The sad part to come out of this revelation is that some of the parents told their children. One of the children told my daughter. She was heart broken. Just as I feared, she believed her mother was about to die. We hadn't told the children. We didn't want them worrying everyday that their parents could die. We wanted to wait until they were older. Unfortunately ignorance about this disease did not allow us the opportunity to have a discussion with our children on our terms. This was a very spiteful and hurtful action.

What this child did to my daughter was wrong. Here was another attack done as a result of the stigma attached to this disease. This required us sitting the oldest children down to teach them about HIV. My Pastor at the time and I had a long discussion, and the conclusion was in spite of our hurt, my daughter and I had to forgive this child. It took time but we forgave her. And if you are reading this we love you. In hindsight, it was a blessing. I believe knowing the status of their parents prepared them for life. Just as we did not take one moment God blessed us to live on this planet for granted, the children also did not take life for granted. They knew more about this disease than most adults.

If we don't start being real about this disease and talk about it to teenagers in our churches, schools, and locker rooms, it's going to continue to spread even faster than it is already spreading to the teenage population. Adults, don't think it is bypassing us. We are on HIV's hit list. No one is talking about it and many are not getting tested. And don't just put this on the church. You have people in church and out of church having sex like there is no tomorrow. Pastors are cheating on their wives. Deacons are cheating on their wives. Deaconesses are cheating on their husbands. Pastors' wives are cheating on their husbands because they know they're cheating with their secretaries or other parishioners. Principals, politicians, and any profession you could possibly name, including people who don't even have a job are included. Sex is running rampant. And guess what? HIV and AIDS are running right along side of it. It's time to stop the madness. If you are sexually active, get tested today. It's too late for me, but some of you might still have a chance.

Now I need to pause here for a minute. If you're reading this and thinking, "Well, I am not having sex outside of my marriage, so I am not sinning against God," remember this. His word says, *"All have sinned and fallen short of the Glory of God." (Romans 3:23 kjv)* There is no big sin and no little sin. If you have told a lie, sin. If you have ever talked about someone, sin. *"When I would do good, evil is always present." (Romans 7:21 kjv)*

There is always some temptation trying to get us to do something wrong. Even Jesus was tempted. *(Matthew 4:1)* So don't you think for one moment that there is not going to be something in your life that will draw you away from God. Stand up in church and talk about the temptations of this world which could also end with the remainder of your life here on earth full of unnecessary sickness and disease.

Tell people that this is not a fun disease to have. I don't want another person on this earth to contract this disease. Aside from the physical anguish, the mental anguish alone is enough to kill you. I was depressed for years and did not realize it. Until I finally faced the mental aspects of this disease, I was not truly set free.

We must realize that some people living with HIV/AIDS feel betrayed by the Church. Some feel unloved, shunned and ostracized. Some may feel unwanted and unwelcome. The few churches they see in the media protesting them, and condemning them to hell unfortunately for many have painted the picture that this is the way all churches feel, although many of us know this is not true. We as ministers of the gospel are bound by the laws of God. But the law of God also commands us to love our neighbor as ourselves. Although we may not agree with the lifestyle of some, we also cannot lump everyone into the category that they are not living a Godly lifestyle because they have contracted this disease.

If someone is living a lifestyle that is contrary to what we have read and the instructions that God has given us in his Holy Word, we still cannot invalidate them, condemn them and not acknowledge that they do not believe what we believe. We have to acknowledge that some individuals may believe this is the way God has made them. This acknowledgement should not pull us out of the character of Christ and feel we need to beat them up and down. We are still bound by his Word to love one another as Christ has loved us. We must continue to let our light shine before men so that they may see our good works and glorify our Father in Heaven. Although there are areas where we may not agree, I can be the friend that Christ has been to me. I can stand with you while you're down, and give you a hand to lift you up.

And to every person who suffers from this disease, don't you feel ashamed by no church folk or any other folks for that matter about what they're going to say about you because you have contracted this disease. Don't concern yourself about anyone who will tear you down because of this disease. In many cases they have done the same things you have. They just may not have caught this disease. They are no better than you, and in God's eyes, we are in the same sinners boat. The only thing you need to know and remember is, *"If we confess our sins, he is faithful and just to forgive us our sins, and to cleanse us from all unrighteousness."* (1John 1:9 kjv) And while you're at it, remember this one too. *"What shall we say then? Shall we continue in sin, that grace may abound? God forbid."* (Romans 6:1-2 kjv)

God is looking for some people who have acknowledged they have done wrong but are making a commitment to him to now do right. And he has promised to those who have truly repented FORGIVENESS!! I put that in caps for a purpose. People will never forgive you. Don't you worry about them. You just worry about God forgiving you. He's the only one who can save your soul. So you walk into any church of your choosing and worship an almighty God who loves you, no matter what you have. I actually look at death differently now because of this disease. No one knows the day or hour when they might die. *(Matthew 24:36)*

Having this disease, I am more focused on death. I've made preparations with my children and family. I've made my peace with God. So when He takes me, I am ready. But what if you're walking around shunning people because they have AIDS? What if you do not want someone to come into your church because they have AIDS? What if you are judging people because of AIDS? What if you are not allowing people with HIV/AIDS to eat off of your plates? You better educate yourself about this disease. Are you gossiping about people behind their backs? Do you think you are better? You better check out your own soul before you start concentrating on whether or not that person is going to hell. *"And why beholdest thou the mote that is in thy brother's eye, but considerest not the beam that is in thine own eye?" (Matthew 7:3 kjv)* Can I get an Amen somebody? Okay!

Sin is sin in God's eye. AIDS is not a sin. Now when we had sex with someone that we weren't married to, that was the sin. When we cheated on our husbands or wives, this was the sin. In this day and age, AIDS might just turn out to be that unfortunate consequence. And, a whole bunch of folks, including church folks, are in the Sex Sin Boat. So let's wake up and jump off the boat, before it sinks.

The church can be a valuable resource in preventing the spread of this disease and ministering to those who are in need. We are instructed to feed the poor, clothe the homeless, and care for the sick and widowed. Well, this disease has left a lot of people poor because they have lost their jobs when employers no longer want to pay their medical bills nor pay them disability. They are left homeless when they can no longer pay their mortgage because they are too sick to hold down a job. They are widowed because the husbands they have been faithful to for 50 years just died from the disease he contracted while sleeping with prostitutes on the side throughout their entire marriage. Now she has the disease and no money because her husband spent all their money on prostitutes. Or maybe the wife just died who gave the husband this disease because she was sleeping with male prostitutes everyday as soon as her husband went to work. He has faithfully worked all his life to provide for his family. Suddenly his wife is dead. She died from AIDS he never knew she had. He has been sick for so long, but did not want to take off from work because he had to provide for his family. Now he can no longer work, his wife is dead, and he doesn't know how he's going to provide for his children.

Sound dramatic? Guess what? In this day and age, this is exactly what is happening. Unnecessary drama is befalling families over what? Sex? There is no sex in this world that's so good that I'm willing to lose my life, family, home, job, and children over. Give up everything is this world, that I have spent a lifetime building? I don't think so! Trust me, there is not one sexual encounter worth it!

Can the church be a resource? Can we step up and stop criticizing and go tell someone of the healing power of Jesus Christ? Can we meet the needs of the people? The church has the resources right in their midst. We have parishioners who are doctors, nurses, medical assistants, health professionals, public health workers, teachers, scientists, laborers and just plain workers, wanting to know how they can help. We have the buildings, classrooms, and space.

As a church the first thing we have to focus on is how God requires us to treat all people, regardless if we agree or disagree with their way of living, thinking or what they believe. We have a commandment that has been given directly to the people of God, which is:

"A new command I give you: Love one another. As I have loved you, so you must love one another. By this all men will know that you are my disciples, if you love one another." (John 13: 34-35 kjv)

"For God so loved the WORLD, that he gave his only begotten Son, that whosoever believeth in him should not perish, but have everlasting life." (John 3:16 kjv)

How then should we treat those living with HIV/AIDS? It makes it a lot easier if we Love them as God loves them. Unconditionally. Acknowledge that our past way of protesting, shunning, gossiping about them, rejecting and judging hasn't made us look too good as a group of people who will be known for the love we have one to another.

Another thing we have to do is acknowledge that we are not a perfect people. *"All have sinned and come short of the Glory of God." (Romans 3:23 kjv)* Be real with people about the ways we have messed up in this world. Acknowledge that we would have been horrified if there was someone protesting outside of our homes or workplace about everything we have done that someone may disagree with or believe is wrong. Treat people as you would want to be treated. We can let people know there was a time in our life that God was not too pleased with the way we lived.

There are many ways that churches can help. First we need to begin to educate our congregations on the ways we can and cannot catch this disease. We can hold seminars or workshops. As people understand this disease they will be less likely to shun or treat people in a negative manner, such as not wanting to hug someone. Not wanting them to eat off your plates or use your utensils. Not wanting them to use your bathroom. Not wanting to invite them into your homes, or not wanting to go into their home. This type of behavior is clearly done by people who are uneducated about the ways this disease can be transmitted.

Also in the education process, we can establish with our congregation that some of their risky behavior of being sexually active without using condoms can place them at risk of contracting this disease. And that using condoms may or may not protect them because they can break. We cannot be in denial that the entire single population of our congregation is being abstinent. So let's get real and educate people about all the various types of ways in which you can contract the disease.

In these education sessions, you can invite representatives from agencies such as Action AIDS and Philadelphia Fight to inform the congregation on all the services available for people living with HIV. These are agencies in Philadelphia, but look for agencies in your communities. This way people who are infected can receive vital information, without coming out about their status, for fear of being shunned or treated in a hateful or judgmental manner. Most of these agencies offer really vital services. Many people living with this disease are not aware of these services because they have not told anyone they are living with the disease. If they are in a forum that's not specifically for people living with this disease they may be more willing to attend. Once in attendance, they can receive this vital information. We can specifically get out where our friends or family members can go for assistance.

We as a congregation have to realize that many people living with HIV/AIDS are suffering alone, some with depression and I believe that many fear the church is the last place they will be accepted. They have seen how people are treated and protested on the news by the Christian community, so they feel this is the last place that they can go to receive assistance. We have to let our members know that they are worshipping in a safe place. That not only do they have God who has never left them nor forsaken them, but we have resources available, where you will not be judged. Let them know they can seek professional mental care without fear of judgment. We can have a designated trustworthy professional who is already working with the HIV/AIDS community which works under a statue of confidentiality. This person can be with an agency, or we may have professionals already as members as our congregation. The number is given to the entire congregation so that individuals can call for one-on-one confidential counseling. No one will know they have called, but the person receives the help they need.

We can hold health fairs. Many churches have large fellowship halls. During these workshops we can offer all types of health services. Blood pressure screening, diabetes testing, and of course free confidential anonymous HIV testing. People will have secured testing done, and only they will know the results. Offer this service because one of the major reasons that this disease is spreading is that many people are sexually active, and do not know their status. If we offer resources at our places of worship for these groups of individuals, we must find ways to let the HIV/AIDS community know what services are available. There are food banks, clothing banks, rental or mortgage assistance, job assistance, etc. We can always reach this community by reaching out to the agencies that serve them and in turn, we become God's agency that's serving them.

Educate our congregation on the population that has the fastest growing rates of increase in HIV/AIDS. There has been an increase in the number of African American teens, African American women, Latino population and now our senior population is also being infected.

Be willing to open our doors to speakers who are living with this disease to come in and openly speak with the congregation about how they contracted the disease and what it has been like to live with this disease. Ask them how the church has made them feel. Let the speaker know they can come without fear of judgment and let the congregation know for many of us, but for the grace of God there goes I.

As a body of Christ come together and let the HIV/AIDS community know that we seek their forgiveness for the way we have treated them in the past. We have not treated them with the love of God. And for that we are sorry. We may not agree in many areas, but we do agree that we must Love one another. And we must do unto others as we would have done unto us.

We can set up classes to teach and educate using the members right in our midst to facilitate these classes. Many of these members are just looking for an area where their gifts, talents and education can be used to benefit mankind. They are not looking to be paid. We can set up this huge kitchen God has blessed us with to feed the hungry. We have space to set up areas where clothes can be donated, for needy families to come and be clothed. We are eligible to receive grants to help the homeless find shelter, and not just any shelter, but one where love, kindness, gentleness, patience, meekness, and self control run rampant. Stop judging people with AIDS and look at what God requires of us:

(Galatians 5:16-26 kjv) "16So I say, live by the Spirit, and you will not gratify the desires of the sinful nature. 17For the sinful nature desires what is

contrary to the Spirit, and the Spirit what is contrary to the sinful nature. They are in conflict with each other, so that you do not do what you want. 18But if you are led by the Spirit, you are not under law. 19The acts of the sinful nature are obvious: sexual immorality, impurity and debauchery; 20idolatry and witchcraft; hatred, discord, jealousy, fits of rage, selfish ambition, dissensions, factions 21and envy; drunkenness, orgies, and the like. I warn you, as I did before, that those who live like this will not inherit the kingdom of God. 22But the fruit of the Spirit is love, joy, peace, patience, kindness, goodness, faithfulness, 23gentleness and self-control. Against such things there is no law. 24Those who belong to Christ Jesus have crucified the sinful nature with its passions and desires. 25Since we live by the Spirit, let us keep in step with the Spirit. 26Let us not become conceited, provoking and envying each other."

Don't sit there with a drink in your hand, getting drunk while telling someone, "How are we going to stop those people with AIDS from coming into our church?" Or you become conceited thinking you are better than others and when the meeting is over, you go meet up with someone on the side.

We as the church stand in judgment over individuals because of the way in which they have contracted this disease. We treat them differently because of their sexual orientation. We want to hold up signs and protest and tell them they are going to hell. But I'm thinking it's time to hold up signs and protest ourselves. Every time we do something wrong or make a mistake, get out a sign and protest yourself. Then maybe we will understand what it feels like to have someone protest against the things you do.

Okay, people want to protest sexual sins. Do you know how many people in this world who are having sex with someone they are not married to? Now let's make it more personal. How many people had sex before they were married? I had been having sex since I was a teenager. How many people in this world have ever cheated on their spouse? Would you like signs held up as soon as you leave the hotel reading, "He or she is an adulterer and they are going to hell? They just had sex in the hotel with someone they were not married to."

How many people are living with someone they are not married to? Each time I got married, I lived with my spouse before we were married. I would have been horrified if someone stood outside of my house saying,

"They are not married yet." Would you like someone to stand outside of your house or apartment with signs saying, "This couple is shacking up! They are going to hell." *"All have sinned and come short of the Glory of God," (Romans 3:23 kjv)* which means everyone in church has committed a sin at some point. The scriptures say we sin daily. So who am I to stand in judgment over the sins of another individual, completely forgetting that I am a sinner saved by God's Grace? Who am I to say that the same Grace that God has given me is not deserving to another individual?

As the church, maybe we could love them as Christ has loved us. I don't know--maybe we could let them know that *"God so loved the world that he gave his only begotten son, that who so ever believed in him should not perish, but have everlasting life." (John 3:16 kjv)* Maybe instead of telling them they are sinners, we could tell them we are all sinners. Let them know about our mistakes, and that we require the same forgiveness that everyone requires. I want to share with someone that the command God gave to keep our bodies as a living sacrifice holy and acceptable to God which is our reasonable service, applies to me. I can't judge you for what you have done; I am too busy going to God repenting for what I have done.

As the church, let's wrap our arms around someone who's lonely and in need and tell them that God loves them. Let's touch someone whose family does not want to touch them anymore because they have this disease. If they can't find solace in church, where are they going to find it?

The church can be a valuable resource. Let us step up to the plate and do something good. We can reach millions of people every Sunday. Get out of the closet and do what is right in the sight of God. Stop this thing before it reaches your kids or your grandkids. I am HIV positive so I can say it; I do not want my children or my future grandchildren to contract this disease. I also do not want you, or your children to contract this disease. Take my word for it, it's no fun. But just in case it's already too late, get tested. Find a doctor to determine if it is time for you to start medication. Take this medication daily. I am living proof that it will help you to live longer.

Churches can set up resources for people to be tested and educated. I am not asking you to promote pre-marital sex. No, I am asking you to do just the opposite. Tell them the truth. It's too much of a risk. Don't do it. Keep your legs closed. Pre-marital sex is a sin against God and trust me, you don't want to suffer the consequence of catching a sexually transmitted disease. If you've already made a mistake, don't worry, everyone in here has made mistakes. We've all sinned and come short of the glory of God. *(Rom. 3:23)* Yes, I've said this scripture over and over again. People tend to focus on someone else's shortcomings, but seem to forget their own shortcomings. The only difference is we have asked God to forgive us. Now repent of your sins and come on over to our resource center. There are some folks over there who will love you as Christ has loved us and provide you with valuable resources to live physically and spiritually in spite of whatever you have done in the past. Everybody in here has a past that doesn't look too pretty, so don't feel bad; you've come just to the right place.

I have had people who I thought were my friends find out that I have HIV and then disappear so fast, you'd think they just performed a magic trick. Then there has been the exact opposite where others who I was not very close with, when they found out, supported me like you would not believe. I was in church one day, came out into the hallway, and caught someone talking about me. She had just said my name and was totally shocked to find me standing right behind her. I still laugh to myself every time I think of that. I would pay money to have a picture of their faces at that exact moment. Now mind you, I am in church. The last place you think this is suppose to happen.

One of the medications I used to take would dry out my mouth and leave white stuff in the corner of my mouth. I had someone look down on me and treat me like I just stepped right out of the drug house and into the hospital to pick up my father. They treated me and my children like crap. I was informed that my children could not go onto the floor, but they watched child after child enter the floor while they had to sit by the door. Instead of offering me a tissue and telling me this stuff was on my mouth, they talked about me like a dog. Some people do not need to be on the nursing staff. You need love and compassion to be a nurse. Unfortunately some have no business being in the profession.

I have found out that there are people who do not want me in their homes because I have HIV. Do you really think you can get it by my walking through your door? You better wake up and educate yourselves about this disease before you or one of your family members go walking through that shut door.

I will never forget hearing about a church in a North Philadelphia neighborhood where the Pastor said no one with AIDS will ever be allowed into their church. I remember feeling so tainted. I am saying to myself I have accepted Jesus Christ as my Lord and Savior. I have changed my life. I have turned everything over to him. But these people still feel I am not good enough to enter their building. In their eyes I am worthless and undeserving of forgiveness.

I refused to accept that. I have read his word and I know he has forgiven me. So if these people do not believe I am worthy of forgiveness, if these people believe I will taint their building, then that's their problem. Get over it. My faith and trust is in God alone. He has forgiven me even if you cannot. I will go wherever I feel like going. I don't need you on my side--I need God on my side. To anyone who feels this way, I believe no one with AIDS wants to go into a church where they are not welcomed.

I cannot imagine that Jesus himself would want to even go into that church. What if Jesus is with a lost soul who he is walking hand-in-hand with to bring to his alter? I guess Jesus would have to by pass your church since the child of God, His holy spirit is with, is not welcome. Hmmm, let's see, the people Jesus hung around included the thief who was hung on the cross with Jesus. The sick he healed. The poor he fed. The lame he healed to walk again. The lepers with disease he healed. I will stick with Jesus. You can keep all empty buildings, void of the Holy Spirit. I will just hang out where the true and living God, who loves unconditionally, dwells. This really does leave me with a pressing question: If Jesus is coming back for a church without a spot or wrinkle and you have banned groups of people from coming into your building, would that be considered a spot or wrinkle?

"You, however, are controlled not by the sinful nature but by the Spirit, if the Spirit of God lives in you. And if anyone does not have the Spirit of Christ, <u>he does not belong to Christ</u>. (Romans 8:9 kjv)

Trust me, just stick with Jesus, and you will be just fine. He will lead you and guide you in all truth. He will lead you to the house of God with those folks who truly belong to God, because God lives in them. I remember being so upset when I first heard about this church. I wanted to write letters and tell them about themselves. My Pastor at the time said, "Darlene, don't worry about them. God will take care of them. They have to answer to God for what they say and do. They have to answer to God for how they have treated one another. You just focus on your relationship with God." That was good and sound advice. Thank you Pastor.

"A new command I give you: Love one another. As I have loved you, so you must love one another. By this all men will know that you are my disciples, if you love one another." (John 13: 34-35 kjv)

If this disease has taught me nothing else, it has taught me tolerance. You may not agree with many people, but in spite of that you must love them. God requires us to love them. Care for them. Be careful how you treat people; it just might be you one day who finds yourself in need.

I wrote a poem after I read that article. Writing has always been a way for me to channel my anger. I found this poem healing to me when people have treated me wrong just because I have this disease. I hope it will help others.

Darlene King

SET APART

I awoke this morning with a disease
A disease that couldn't happen to me
This happens to others, not to me
I thought I was set apart from this disease
I found myself in a new group, in a group
    I didn't choose
Made up of babies, children and the like
Regular people from all walks of life
As I examined the friends in my group
I realized they also didn't choose
Choose to be set apart, discarded, or so I thought
But then came a Savior, from out of nowhere
To give us something we could share
He told us we were set apart
But, not apart as we thought
We were set apart, to be used, to his Glory,
    if we choose
He let us know that we were special
As were all the children who became his vessel
As I embraced my new found troop
I realized my disease didn't matter in this group
The criteria was so simple
To follow his plan of redemption

HIV Infected by Her Cheating Pastor Husband

To Love, Give, Care and Share
And accept those others wouldn't dare
And in the end we'd have a resting place
Where my disease would be erased
So regardless of what disease, fear or phobia you face
Be assured you have a resting place
Just be careful that on your way
You don't discard a vessel God has placed
So when you choose to be set apart
Be set apart with God in your thoughts

Chapter 7
How Did I End Up with the Title?

I found out I was HIV positive by giving blood to the Red Cross. I always donated blood when they held blood drives at my place of employment. On this particular occasion, a few weeks after giving blood, I received a letter from the Red Cross. The letter stated that I was HIV positive, and I should contact my doctor as soon as possible. I was devastated.

The letter said to contact all the people you have been with in the last 10 years. All tested negative except my future husband and Pastor. He kept saying I don't need a test. Then he claimed he finally went and it was positive. I later found out that he already knew from the moment I first called him that he was HIV positive. He also knew of others he had infected with HIV. He went into what I now know as fake, I love you. "I have always loved you. I want to spend the rest of my life with you. Let's get married. I will take care of you."

Anyway, we decided to get married and commit the rest of our lives together. Little did I know how one sided that commitment was. In all my wildest dreams and goals for my life, I never once said to myself, "I want to become a First Lady." Who sits around and thinks of this as a goal for themselves? Well I found out the hard way that a lot of women are sitting in churches trying to obtain that exact goal. Well, I say be careful what you ask for; you just might get it. Personally, my experience has been that you can take my title and keep it for life. I never want to hold it again! I have never seen anything so ridiculous until I witnessed women throwing themselves at a man just because he is the Pastor of the church. Right in front of my face, they would flirt with my husband. There were times I was so sick of him, under my breath I would be saying, "Take him, free me from this mess."

If they only knew. You think he told these women he was HIV positive? No he did not. He had the nerve to tell me about one of the women who invited him over. And the first thing out of my mouth was, "Did you tell her about the HIV?" His response was, "No." I said tell her and see if she still wants you to come over. He never mentioned her again. Periodically I would ask questions about the lady because she all of a sudden stopped attending church. Of course his answer was that he hadn't spoken with her. I would say to myself, "Too bad. I guess he won't be running off with her."

This was at the point where I was so sick of the deception. I was in this marriage for almost 12 years and was in and out of relationships with him since the age of 12. We attended middle school and high school together. Ladies, I know I learned the hard way. But most likely if they have lied to you from age 12 to 44, they are going to be lying until you die. Don't wait as long as I did. The longer you wait, that much more of yourself will be lost in the process.

When I got married, I really thought I was marrying a person who had been my friend for most of my life. We had dated off and on for years. Now we had contracted this disease and we were committing the rest of our lives together to be there for one another when we got sick. I should have known all bets were off when the first cheating I found out about was three months after being married. This resulted in our youngest son being born on the exact day of our first wedding anniversary. From that point on, it became a quarterly exercise of him getting caught, making up, and me leaving or about to leave. You get my drift.

Twelve years of this mind you. One year towards the end, after years of celebrating Mother's Day I was told, "Oh, I didn't know if I should buy you anything for Mother's Day since you are not my mother." Oh, I just have 2 kids and 6 step-children. I think I should be allowed to celebrate Mother's Day. You celebrate you, every moment of every day of every year.

Now before I suggest the following, I want to first let you know that marriage is an institution, ordained by God. I fully believe in the institution of marriage. You should at all cost do what you can to save your marriage. *(Hebrews 13:4 kjv) "Marriage should be honored by all, and the marriage bed kept pure, for God will judge the adulterer and all the sexually immoral."* But more importantly, we should at all cost live in our marriages in obedience to God by doing exactly what he requires in our marriage, which is keep the sanctity of our marriage, pure and holy unto God. If we choose to do something other than what God requires, then we have chosen to break the covenant agreement we made with God, in stating our vows before him.

Although if your husband is the Pastor and you are the First Lady of the Church, and you have been told any of the following stories, it may be time to run.

Wait a minute, let me rephrase. If you are a man or woman, and you are in a relationship, and you have been told any of the following stories, RUN. You will say, "I would never stay under those circumstances." And you would be right to declare such a statement. Because the result of staying under the following circumstances will be much therapy required. (Side bar: Therapy will be covered in another chapter.)

Interesting Q & A over many years

Question: "You are the Pastor, how can you be going to strip clubs?"

Answer: "I am an undercover agent for the FBI and the DEA. My friend, who is a cop, knew I had street cred, and I had to go in for him because he could be identified."

Question: "Where is your paycheck for the undercover work with the FBI and DEA? The mortgage is due; we need the money from this undercover work."

Answer: "Why are you asking me all these questions? You don't believe me? I'll give you his number. You can call him yourself. This is why I don't tell you anything. You don't believe anything I say." Walks out of the room hollering. (Note: Walking away to think of more lies, and you never get a number to call)

(Note to anyone listening. RUN, RUN..........)

Question: "Why is she calling my house saying she is pregnant by you?"

Answer: "She has the wrong number; I don't know who you're talking about."

Question: "The same woman you don't know is calling your cell, beeper, and now she is on the house phone; she wants to speak with you."

Answer: "I don't love her. I only love you. It just happened one time; I'll never do it again."

Question: "Did you forget you don't know her? I can't believe you're still sleeping with women, and even worse, how can you sleep with people without a condom and not tell them you have HIV?"

Answer: "It only happened one time. The condom must have broken. I made a mistake. Please take me back. I'll never do it again. This is just the devil trying to break up our marriage. Satan is trying to come between us and mess up everything we have."

Question: "The Gynecologist said I have another sexually transmitted disease on top of the ones I already have."

Answer: "I want to talk to him. They made a mistake. I have not slept with anyone. I will go down there and prove it. You need to take that test over again. Nothing is wrong with me. There must be something wrong with you."

(Note: RUN, RUN…….. PLEASE RUN)

Question: "This woman keeps calling my house. I pressed *69, and called her house back. Guess what happened. Her answering service is a message you left on her machine. It appears that you have found a good and crazy one this time around. She has changed her answering machine to your voice with a message you left, saying you loved her and that you had a really good time last night. You want to hear it?"

Answer: "No I didn't! I was not with any women!"

Question: "You sure you don't want to hear this?"

Answer: He calls the number and listens to the message. (Note: I wish I had a picture of the look on his face.)

Question: "I thought you didn't know her."

Answer: "I can't believe she did that. She is trying to set me up. I just said that because I wanted her to feel good about herself. I never met her. (4 seconds later) Okay, I did meet her. But it wasn't anything. I can't believe she did that. I am so sorry. I'll never do that again."

Question: "Did you tell her you were HIV positive?"

Answer: "No."

Question: "Why would you want to get someone pregnant?"

Answer: "Because you won't have a baby."

Question: "Have you lost your mind, why would I purposely give my baby HIV?"

Answer: "That doesn't mean anything; you could have a baby if you wanted to."

It was the stupidest thing I had ever heard. I had no response. I just walked out of the room shaking my head. Believe it or not, I was asked again numerous times to have a baby. Ridiculous! I just wanted to smack him! (Run, Run, Run…)

God has a unique way of coming in and settling arguments which should not have been arguments in the first place. I was always thinking why do I have to have these stupid discussions about having another baby; is he crazy? Next thing you know, I am afflicted with fibroid tumors, and I had to have a hysterectomy to have them removed. I was no longer able to conceive children. Talk about God's ways are not our ways. Some things may seem like a tragic event in your life; but they may be the trial that changes your situation for the better. That was the end of the baby discussion.

Thank you, Jesus, for ending that stupid argument. By the way, guess who disappeared and became unreachable while I was in the hospital? And when he finally showed up at the hospital he did not understand why I was not able to reach him on the cell phone. There was probably no signal.

(Do you see where this is going? There's a signal alright. And the signal reads: RUNNN…)

Oh, the years of stories just like this, from age 12. Every time we broke up, it was because of him messing with other girls. And I always took him back. I will never forget the time we broke up before we eventually got married when I said to him, "I cannot stay with you. You keep sleeping with all these people. You are going to get HIV sleeping with all these people." And based on the timing, he was probably already HIV positive. But unfortunately, I believed by time we got married, and at that point we were both HIV positive, all the sleeping around would end. People please listen: If HIV does not stop someone from sleeping around, believe me, nothing will.

This First Lady thing was on his mind for a long time. He said to me, "I married you because I need a wife that is fit for church." Somebody please tell me-- what in the heck does that mean? I could not believe he said this. I was really worried when he first said it. I think he could tell I was worried because he tried to clean it up. "No, I just mean someone who loves going to church." Yeah, right.

In hindsight, which is the sight I have had to view pretty much my entire life, since he has been in it most of my entire life, there was another meaning in that statement. It gave a glimpse into this quest to one day become a Pastor. And I ended up in this role as First Lady. I don't want to be fit for church. I want to be fit for worship. I want to be fit for the Master's use. I want to be an obedient servant of the most High God. I want to be found worthy of the vocation in which I have been called. I pray daily for God to create in me a clean heart and renew a right spirit in me. I need God to restore me to the joy of my salvation.

I have to constantly ask him to cast me not away from his presence and to take not his Holy Spirit from me. I sin daily--we sin daily. Church for me is a place of solace and a place to forget all the cares of this world. I am at peace in worship. I am at peace in praise. I need the renewal. I need a place to come together with others who have a mind to worship.

In most churches, the wife of the Pastor is called First Lady. I added this point because of an article I read. The writer expressly pointed out that the Pastor's wife is called First Lady, as if he did not realize that this is what they are called in churches all over America. Now the first thing I want to clear up is not to let a few rotten apples spoil the entire batch. We have some wonderful, dedicated men and women of God, who live their lives for Christ. They spend their lives in dedication to serving the flock of people God has placed in their care. They do this with love and devotion that you cannot begin to imagine. These are the majority. There are a small few who do the opposite. But because it is such a scandal when it happens, we sometimes lump everyone into the same category. Well, we cannot. My experience that I share as a First Lady applies only to me. I can only tell you what I felt. I can only tell you what I experienced. I can only tell you this was not a job I asked for, nor would I pick this job for myself. First of all, God has to place you in this job. You must be called by God to become a Pastor and First Lady of a church.

When I took this role, my only goal was to help people, serve God and treat others with the same love and kindness that I would want someone to treat me. And in the beginning of our ministry, we worked so hard together to serve the community. Our focus was on target. We were helping families and youth. We were building a church. Our children were involved and committed because they saw our commitment. But power and sex destroyed everything that was beautiful and good. Women, don't throw yourself at these men in church. If they are going to be disobedient and disrespectful to an all knowing, all powerful God, what kind of respect do you think they will have for you? In the end you will only become just something on the side. And mind you, these days, it's sex, with a possible side of HIV.

I never thought women would just disrespect me right in front of my face while I was sitting in church. There was no care or concern of breaking up my home. What they did not know was he was already doing a great job of destroying our family before they came into the picture. And they sure would not have been so quick to jump in the bed if they knew the HIV side of the story. I hope this makes those of that type of mindset think twice before such an action. Looks can be very deceiving. Titles can be very deceiving. Don't go rushing to hop on someone just because he's a Pastor or holds some other prestigious title. You don't know who or what they have already hopped on. The same respect you would like to receive is the respect you should look to give.

I have watched people whisper in his ears, pass him notes, and sit and purposely pull their dresses up to their knees so their legs would be out. They always needed meetings at my house during the hours that I was at work. They would buy him all sorts of gifts. Some would say degrading things to you to try and make you feel bad about what you are wearing or how you look. But of course this is only being told to you in "love." Yeah right child, please!

That last year, I begged him to leave. I had to stop sleeping with him. He was hanging out in strip clubs again. He was snorting coke, but I didn't find this out until the end. Women were calling our home. He would disappear for days and then come home drunk or high. He got paid on Friday, come home Sunday morning to preach, and leave for another three or four days. His paycheck is now gone. I am struggling to pay all the bills. He is bouncing checks, getting payday loans, but he no longer has direct deposit. So his payday loans would come out of my check deposits before I could pay any bills. Finally, I stopped going to church, and I stopped my children from going. Enough was enough. I know you are thinking enough came and went a long time ago. But you have to come to your own end. And you will know when you have reached that end.

He had promised the time before our last and final split that if things did not work out, he would be the one to leave. Of course, he refused to leave. And I guess he thought I loved that house so much I would never leave. The only thing at that moment that I loved was Jesus Christ, my sanity and the thought of possible peace. After months of begging him to leave, and many last straws, I was set free on September 5, 2003. He called me "stupid" over and over again. He said, "What kind of First Lady are you? You're supposed to stick with me." I said, "Is this really your definition of a Pastor and First Lady?"

We had a beautiful 4 bedroom, 3 bath home which I loved. But after being kicked in the stomach, cursed at and told I married beneath me, I knew it was over. He really thought I would not leave because I loved our house. That house no longer held a speck of sentimental meaning for me. I became disgusted by that house just thinking about the prostitutes and any new diseases I may have contracted. I did not know who or what had come through there while I was at work and the children were at school. You could feel the demons in that house.

I am turning up my face now at the thought of what probably occurred in that house and what additional diseases could have possibly come my way with such risky behavior. The house no longer mattered.

At that moment, I would have given up anything in this world for two minutes of peace. I packed what I could in trash bags and what my two girls could pack. I knew without a shadow of a doubt, I was leaving and never coming back. The house did not matter. Nothing mattered. All I knew was my children and I would never endure this again.

All he could say while I was packing was, "You stupid girl, you stupid girl, you stupid girl." I said,

"Yes, I was, but I am not anymore." And I made the best decision of my entire life the moment I walked out of that door. The result was peace like you would never believe existed!

We had a written agreement of who would receive which items from the home. He went down my side of the list and destroyed everything I was supposed to receive. He cut up the couch with a butcher knife. When I saw the couch with the butcher knife still sitting on there I said to myself, "That couch is sliced as if he were trying to slice me." I was convinced I got out just in time. All of the glass and mirrors that adorned the bedroom set were broken. Things I loved disappeared from the house. The house was trashed from top to bottom, and then after the water, electricity, and everything else was cut off, he just left.

I was now responsible for the house. He called and said, "It broke your heart to see all your stuff torn up, didn't it?" I told him no, actually it did not. My first thought when I walked into my front door was this is the stupidest thing anyone could have done. He called me stupid. It does not get any stupider than this. I cannot believe I married the stupidest man on the planet. This stuff did not just belong to me. It also belonged to you, idiot. I am looking around saying to myself, "Now this is what you call stupid. Did it ever cross your mind to just sell it? Hmmm, I have no money. I have lost my job. Maybe I'll sell the furniture and the items from the house, to try and get back on my feet?" Duhh... Trust me. You can replace material things. They are just that, things. Nothing in this life is more important than your soul, your children, your family and your life.

Later I found out that crack was the culprit. Just like I said before, it's one of the worst drugs out there. It will strip you of all human dignity and leave you destitute like you cannot begin to imagine. There is no sex and there is no drug worth turning your back on God. God requires more, and God deserves more. And you deserve more for yourself.

(2 Peter 2:21-22 kjv) "It would have been better for them not to have known the way of righteousness, than to have known it and then to turn their backs on the sacred command that was passed on to them. Of them the proverbs are true: A dog returns to its vomit, and a sow that is washed goes back to her wallowing in the mud."

When someone focuses on the mistakes and downfall of man or spiritual leaders, it can sometimes destroy his or her faith. I thank God every day that this did not destroy the faith of our children. And, I beg of you, do not allow what someone else may do to destroy your faith nor have you turn your back on God. If someone makes a bad choice, then he has to live with his choices. You choose to do what is right. What others have done has nothing to do with you. Keep your eyes on God. Man can sometimes fail. God never fails. If you have been hurt in church or by a spiritual leader, make up your mind today that I am going back to GOD.

Now hear what I am saying. I did not say I am going back to church, a building or structure. That is just that--a building. I am going where I can freely worship God in spirit and in truth. I am going where I am welcome to come as I am. I am going back to God. I am going back to the place where my soul exploded with peace. I am going back to where I experienced unspeakable joy. I am going back to where unending praise leapt from my lips. I am going back to where I freely danced out of myself. That can only happen on the inside. We are the church, and God lives inside of US. Do not forsake the fellowship of the saints. God has a place of true worship just for you. Ask him to help you find that place.

(John 4:23 kjv) "But the hour cometh, and now is, when the true worshippers shall worship the Father in spirit and in truth: for the Father seeketh such to worship him."

(Hebrews 10:25 kjv) "Not forsaking the assembling of ourselves together, as the manner of some is; but exhorting one another: and so much the more, as ye see the day approaching."

Getting back to this place was not easy. I was so hurt and so embarrassed. I never wanted to step my feet into church again. All I wanted to do was curl up in a corner and die. At that moment, it was the most devastating thing that had happened to me in my entire life. I had made up my mind that I was never going to church again. Like I've said, our plans are not his plans. Our thoughts are not his thoughts. Our way is not his way. God placed people in my life who had a determination they were not going to let me go until I received my breakthrough. A mindset was in these individuals, and a determination that only God can place on their hearts was directed at my family.

Our new Pastor, who took over the leadership, prayed and called me constantly to make sure I would not give up on God. The women of our church wrapped their arms around my children and I and wouldn't let us go. They called daily. They prayed daily. God lead me to return. If I missed a Sunday, they were on my phone. When I looked up, they were at my mother's door. In them I saw a living example of how God requires us to minister to others in their time of need. Still today, I pull from this experience when I reach out to help others. Stand firm until your breakthrough comes, and like Jacob, don't let go of God until he blesses you. And we, who are strong in the faith, use every opportunity given to hold our brothers and sisters up, and not let them go until their change comes. My prayer has always been that all of us who are affected by this disease would have someone sent by God to minister to us and pray us through during our time of need.

(Genesis 32 kjv) "24And Jacob was left alone; and there wrestled a man with him until the breaking of the day. 25And when he saw that he prevailed not against him, he touched the hollow of his thigh; and the hollow of Jacob's thigh was out of joint, as he wrestled with him. 26And he said, Let me go, for the day breaketh. And he said, I will not let thee go except thou bless me."

Chapter 8
<u>Pain Like You Wouldn't Believe</u>

There are people who have truly experienced some really severe pain. My feeling is that I did not experience pain until the following happened to me. You have a Charlie horse in your thighs. It has contracted and become hard as rocks. The rocks are now being pushed through your veins, and your heart feels like it is about to burst out of your chest.

Let me give you another example. Imagine that someone is pushing a baby through the veins in your thighs, but there is no opening, so it is now being forced open. That is the only way I can explain HIV neuropathy and the nerve pain I experienced in my thighs and legs. You can also get this from diabetes, so maybe mine is worse because I have a combination of them both.

All I can tell you is that I vividly remember the first attack. I mean attack because it happened when I was asleep, and I was jarred out of my sleep as if I were being attacked. This pain had me convinced that I was about to die. It was the closest thing at that point which I had experienced which led me to believe I would die at that moment. All I could do was scream and pray at the same time. Now you start having these attacks over and over again. When you fall asleep, your thighs and legs also fall asleep. And worse, you go to the doctors and hospitals, and they cannot figure out what is wrong with you. This pain is in my hips, thighs, legs, and feet. The doctors try all kinds of medication and tests, but nothing works. I am put in physical therapy. Four days before my last day of physical therapy, I am hit from behind in a car accident. Now my face, ear, jaw, neck, shoulders, arms, upper, mid, and lower back are in excruciating pain.

Did you ever hear the expression "Tore up from the floor up?" I am literally torn up from the floor up. Now, there is no part of my body that is not hurting. I lay there like a stiff board. Any movement sends screeching pain through my body. It sometimes feels like there is a three-foot-long needle being pushed from my butt to my neck.

Now this, of course, is happening after leaving my life of misery, and I am thinking, "Okay God, you say *'All things work together for good, to them who Love*

God, to them who are the called according to your purpose.' (Romans 8:28 kjv)" I am lying in bed, unable to move, talking to God, saying, "Okay God, show me the purpose." I talk to God like this all the time. He's my best friend. He knows everything, so I have no problem being real with him. I am saying, "God there could not possibly be a reason for me to be in this much pain." To my dismay, my pain only got worse.

In one of my many visits to the hospital, and after several months and tests later, I found out that I had neuropathy. This is along with my kidneys failing, an irregular heartbeat, a heart murmur, lungs that weren't at full function, herniated discs, a jaw out of line, ear pain that never went away, constant sinus infections, high blood pressure, constant back pain, and an immune system that catches any and every germ that I come in contact with.

This was the point in my life when I fell apart. I trusted God. I believed in God. I knew God would heal me in His time and in His way. But I couldn't handle another thing happening to me. At this point, I fell apart like never before. My physical pain was now laced with mental pain and anguish. I went into depression. Let me rephrase. I finally acknowledged that I had been suffering from depression for some time, and I needed help.

Chapter 9
Wake Up!
You're Suffering from Depression

(Romans 8:26 kjv) "In the same way, the Spirit helps us in our weakness. We do not know what we ought to pray for, but the Spirit himself intercedes for us with groans that words cannot express."

It has been almost impossible to place the feelings of depression into words. Here is my feeble attempt to try. I found myself in the grips of loneliness. Vengeance and anger poured from me like beads of sweat. Self-loathing became my middle name. The presence of evil encamped all around me. Trust escaped me. Hostility became my countenance. Depression like you can never imagine was destined to overtake me for a lifetime. Depression grips you and distorts every point of view. Everything spelled discouragement and gloom, and dejection filled a downhearted soul. I cried enough tears to soak a pillow. I slept enough to dent a mattress. There was no chance of hope. This is just a small glimpse into what I felt. Believe me, it was worse than this.

One of my best friends said to me, "Darlene, I thank God that you didn't lose your mind. Most people who have gone through what you have gone through would have lost their mind." And I thank God too, that I didn't lose my mind. There are others who have ended up in a mental institution. But there were truly times I thought I would completely lose it. I was only kept by his grace and mercy. The isolation and devastation you feel at the news of HIV can hit you like a ton of bricks. So many emotions are running through your head. You don't have a chance to think. Your brain feels like it is going to shut down, and the only option you feel like you have at that moment is to just close out everything. You don't want to think. You don't want to make any decisions. You don't want to discuss what you are feeling. You don't want anyone to know. All you want is to shut out the entire world, curl up in a corner, and die.

I have read a lot of articles and seen a lot of television stories about depression. But I want to talk to the people who have experienced this for themselves and the family members who are struggling to understand and are having to suffer alongside them.

I would also like to talk to people who have dedicated their lives to treating people with this illness or anyone who has compassion and would like to know how they can help.

I know one thing--if someone comes to me and tells me, "You are a Christian, just get over it, and get yourself together," that will make me want to slap someone. Unless you have been through what I have, and are dealing with the issues I face, don't tell me to get myself together. You don't have to wonder everyday if you're going to live long enough to see your children graduate from high school and college. You do not have to wonder if you will ever see your children marry and someday have children of their own. Do you have to wonder if you will have the strength to play with your grandchildren? These are real issues for people living with HIV--these issues and countless others. Until you have to live it with me daily, don't give me any stupid comments on depression.

To those who suffer, use every resource that is available to you. Do not let anyone discourage you from any form of treatment you choose. If it is helping you, and it is not going to kill you and you are an adult, embrace the treatment that will help you. I waited too long to get help. And once I finally made the decision to get help, I realized I needed this help a long time ago.

I had held on to too many issues and suffered in silence. By the time I starting seeing a therapist, I thought I was going to explode. But God blessed me with the most compassionate, loving and friendliest young lady you will ever meet. I pray that your experience will be as pleasant as mine.

I had a hard time telling my family that I was depressed. I thought if they knew how much mental pain and anguish I was in, this would only break their hearts and want them to seek revenge. But I believe the scripture which reads, *"Vengeance is mine; I will repay, saith the Lord." (Romans 12:19 kjv)* So I held it all in. I never let them know what I was truly feeling. I never let them see me cry. But this young lady gave me an opportunity to talk, cry, and release so much pain. I realized until I released all the hurt, I could never forgive and be forgiven. So I poured my pain onto the pages. With every word I write I am releasing the pain from my spirit.

Some people need medication to help them. I needed medication, and for me, it helped immensely.

In my depression, I would stay in bed for days and just cry. The moment my children left the house, I would just cry. I couldn't eat. I was constantly nauseous. My self-esteem had deteriorated to the point where I loathed myself. I blamed myself for everything that had happened in my life. I beat myself up unmercifully. I felt unworthy and worthless. Misery became my days. Sleep was the only thing I wanted because then I didn't have to think about my life. I was convinced my life was over.

Memory is a funny thing. Most of my memory is gone. The things I have forgotten are numerous. There are so many things that I just cannot remember. But all the bad, demeaning, hurtful things will not leave my head. I could not tell you the names of my teachers nor any of the students I attended elementary school with. But I can tell you how horrible these children treated me. I was bussed to another school against my will and I hated every moment. Parents, ask your children if they want to be bussed to another school. For years I felt, "Did I do something bad to deserve being shipped over here with these horrible people?" I can't tell you what I wore yesterday. But ask me how something horrible made me feel, and I will be able to describe this to you in exact detail.

The thought of me killing myself crossed my mind so many times. I was like, "Be done with it already!" I am here only because of God's grace and mercy, and my children. If I didn't have children, I don't know where I would be. No, if I didn't have children I know I would not be here. As fast as the thoughts of suicide came into my head, I would see my daughters, and just that fast, the thought would leave.

When I found out that one of my daughter's kidneys was not forming as it should, then I actually felt pain in my chest. It was bad enough facing death. The thought that something would happen to any of my children was enough to make me lose my mind. I kept a brave face in front of her, but by myself, I prayed and cried like never before. I couldn't stop crying. I couldn't wait for those kids to walk out the door, and I just dropped to the floor and wailed.

It started with a lump on her chest. From the moment I saw it, a lump welled up in my stomach, which did not leave for days. We rushed to the doctors, and after the test they determined that her kidneys were not forming properly. But they said the lump was just her bone structure. I am in pieces. All I could think was can anything else possibly happen?

As bad as my world fell apart, my children stayed strong. They stayed on the honor roll. I recall myself watching them, but they were watching me. I had to get better for their sakes.

My daughter announced that she was dropping out of college to get a job, so she can help pay the bills. I told her, "Never!" I didn't care what happened to me, but she had to finish school. With all that I had lost, her leaving school would have devastated me. I had to find a way for her to stay in school. And only by God's grace, was she able to stay in school.

I truly thank God for the young lady who became my therapist. This young lady allowed me to be myself and talk. I just needed someone else in the room who would listen and not judge. I needed this escape. I began to crave this escape. The more I let go, the better I felt. God, therapy and medication healed me.

I know I have said it, but I truly thank God for my therapist. When I was with her she made me feel she truly didn't see HIV. She saw Darlene. She saw a woman in pain and wanted to help her through that pain. I was free to open up and share my most intimate hurts. This person cared about what I had to say and wanted to help me. Twelve years of what I could not speak about to my spouse poured out. I lived in a marriage with a disease I wasn't allowed to discuss. I went into this marriage under a one-sided false pretense. I believed that I had a partner on the same page with me. We were going to work out how to live with this disease together. We were going to figure out who would raise our children if something happened to us. There was supposed to be a plan on how we were going to help each other die. But once that wedding was over, I was shut down at every conversation. "I don't want to talk about it." This was the only response I received. Therapy freed me from twelve years of hurt and disappointment. I was free to talk. This is what I craved and never knew it.

Many may choose not to take medication. I say do what you have to do to heal. Don't spend years in denial that you have a problem. Do not give up on yourself. You are special. You are important. The people who really matter have your best interest at heart. To this day, I still have my bouts. I still have my moments. I just pray and trust God. I put my focus on him. You can and will come out on top. Speak your healing into existence, and by faith, believe you will receive it. Just as you embraced the sorrow, embrace right now your deliverance.

I have too much to be done to wallow in sorrow. I heard a great preacher on television in a sermon say, "When sorrows like sea billows roll, there's still work to be done." I am telling you--get in the word, over the word, under the word, and around the word until your change comes. God can and will give you exactly what you need, when you need it.

The word can be found everywhere you turn--on the radio and on television. Turn on a TBN broadcast, or The Word Network; early in the morning, or late at night. I will turn on that television or radio, and you couldn't tell me they weren't talking directly to me. There would be a sermon on a topic speaking specifically about a situation I am facing at that moment. Diligently seek the word of God, and God will give you exactly what you need at that moment.

I opened this chapter with what depression felt like. I am going to try to put into words what it felt like when God's Love pulled me from the grips of despair. Love oozed through my very pores and wrapped me into its grips like a new scarf. I was surrounded with comfort like a robe adorned with the garment of praise.

I felt like I was being caressed in new silk pajamas. This love stretched and felt unending. The essence of tender passion of a first true love filled my room. The urge to bask in the pleasure of peace and joy engulfed me. I felt like I had found a treasure like no other treasure that has been found. Immense infatuation filled me. I felt unworthy, yet I was reassured that through Christ I have been made worthy. I felt undeserving of this Love, but God brought back to my remembrance that it is not because of what I have done, but it is the gift of God, not of works lest any man should boast. Mercy surrounds me, love embraced me, joy overwhelmed me, and hope engulfed me. I truly felt the power to tell mountains to move. My blinded eyes were opened.

I was immediately washed whiter than snow. I knew instantaneously that I would never be left nor forsaken ever again. Perfect peace enveloped the room. Power, love, and a sound mind were deposited in me. Hope was for the asking. Compassion and patience was plentiful. I knew beyond a shadow of a doubt that God would look beyond my faults and see my needs. I felt the worth that was far above rubies. Surely there was a tremendous cost I must have to pay for this new found freedom. There was no cost; there was no fee. Jesus Christ was the ultimate sacrifice for my sins. Jesus paid the cost in full for my redemption. All I needed to do was accept him with my whole heart. Take every care, every concern, and truly turn each situation completely over to him.

The light of Christ burned like a torch in my soul. I truly was transformed by the renewing of my mind. I did not see my situation as it had been viewed in my mind in the past. My thoughts were now on God and now on all that was good. I was able to think on those things that were pure, think on those things that were good, and think on those things that were kind. I was given new life through Jesus Christ our Lord. I had a new outlook, and the work before me became clear. I was set free. He whom the son sets free, is free indeed. I am trying as best as I can to describe my transformation. I just cannot find the words needed to describe Christ's unconditional love that he bestows on his children. Just know that Christ loves you like no other, and that he cares for every aspect of your life. You can trust him with all. Another person's definition of who I am does not matter. I will define who I am. I am a child of the King and He loves me unconditionally.

"I am the door: by me if any man enters in, he shall be saved and shall go in and out, and find pasture. The thief cometh not, but for to steal, and to kill, and to destroy: I am come that they might have life, and that they might have it more abundantly. I am the good shepherd: the good shepherd giveth his life for the sheep." (John 10:9-11 kjv)

Chapter 10

<u>Who Am I Really?</u>

"First Lady" is not the title I would choose for myself. If I am allowed to pick a title, I would like to be called "A Grateful Servant of God." If not that, then call me Mom, Aunt Di, Ms. Darlene, or just simply Darlene. Those are the only titles that fit for me.

I have worked my entire life. My first job was a papergirl. This is where I learned if you truly worked hard, you can achieve anything. A contest was held to sign up a certain amount of customers and if we achieved our goal, we could win a new 10-speed bike. I served papers to three blocks. By the end of that contest, I think I had just about every household on my three blocks signed up to receive the paper. I won that 10-speed bike. You couldn't tell me anything. Working like a dog became my name. I worked for almost 30 years. Nights, weekends, overtime--it didn't matter; I would take it.

Most of my jobs involved customer service. I loved working with people. If someone had a problem that I could fix, I would go out of my way to help him or her receive any benefits he or she was entitled to receive. It bothered me when I couldn't help someone. I would lie in bed and think about the people I was not able to help, and what other departments I could contact in the morning that may be able to help. I could never let it go. People would say, "Don't take this work home with you." I never figured out how not to take it home with me.

I was previously married. I have two of the most wonderful daughters God could bless a person with, and I have wonderful step-children. My girls would do anything for their mother. But these days I know most of what they do is worry about me. One graduated from college and has just returned. The other is currently enrolled in college. They quite often ended up on the honor roll. I try to tell them all the mistakes I have made because I want them to make better choices. I don't want them to work all their lives only to end up destitute. I am so proud of them. They are the reason that I love working with children. I think I missed the boat when I did not pursue becoming a teacher.

Once I rededicated my life to Christ at age 30, I fully committed myself to serving God. I worked in all areas of youth ministry. Anything that involved kids, my hand was the first in the air. I plunged into ministry just as I had plunged into my jobs. I always tried new ideas and tried to add new programs that the kids would enjoy. If they loved rap music, then we would do gospel rap. They loved the drill team, so I was like, let's step for Christ. Many may not have agreed, but my theory is get them involved in what they love. And in most cases, what they love can be used to glorify God. I always tried to help others and treat people with kindness. This is why I believe God has blessed me to receive help from the most wonderful people you ever want to meet.

After years of working and helping others, I was now in a position where I was too sick to work. It was devastating to work for so many years, making a decent income, always being able to provide for your family, and then wake up one day with nothing. One of the saddest moments after losing everything was the day my daughter's period came on, and she came to me and said she needed pads. The pain I felt at not being able to provide my child's basic needs left me in utter agony. I moved in with my mother and father once I fled from my home. After the accident, I couldn't work. I had to use all my savings just for my children and I to survive. I signed up with various agencies to receive help. This is when I began to meet some of the kindest and most compassionate people you could ever meet. They helped us with resources to get back on our feet. I believe if you treat others right in life, kindness is what will come back to you. From my case manager, to the welfare department, to housing agencies, even representatives at Family Court, I was always greeted with love and kindness. God blessed us with a place to live when we had no money to get a place. God blessed us with food, clothing, and medicine. He blessed my daughter to stay in college when we had no money to keep her in college. Every area where there was a need in our life, God provided a way to meet this need.

I tell everyone who has tested positive to sign up with agencies which will provide you with a case manager. Do not let pride get in the way of receiving a blessing. I pray that you are blessed to receive someone as compassionate as I had. They are there to help you. You may be afraid to let someone know you have this disease, but if you don't, you will never receive help that you may desperately need. My case manager helped me find resources I never knew existed. This is when I began to see that all things truly do work together for the good, for those who love God and are called according to his purpose. I was constantly in the doctor's office, welfare office, and other agencies.

I would always meet women and men that suffered my same plight. Some I would tell my stories, and many would tell me theirs. I found myself praying right in the doctor's office or the welfare office. I was meeting and ministering to people in all walks of life. It was nothing for me to be talking to someone and just stop and start praying right on the corner. God began to use every experience that I had suffered to help someone who may be suffering in the same situation. I had done it all and been through it all, so most of the people I met, I could relate to their issue from personal experience. The nonsense ended in my life when God was ready for it to end.

My Pastor sent me to study to become an Evangelist. I remember him asking what my title will become once I finish school. I said, "I don't need a title; Darlene will do just fine." I had a wonderful friend remind me about a time that someone stole my car. I had the kids up in the middle of the night praying for the person who took the car. I explained to them that we can't be mad at him, because he is a lost soul. When someone goes through life thinking he can just take what he wants, it's only a matter of time before he ends up in jail, or even worse--dead. And if the latter comes before they have a chance to turn their lives around, their soul will be lost for all eternity. We can get another car, but he cannot get another soul. So we prayed, and then went back to sleep. That was all I could think of to do. I never gave it a lot of thought, but my friend always reminds me of the great example it set for the children. I thank God because I always want to be a great example for my children, and for that matter, all children. Oh I make a lot of mistakes, but I try to just do what is right and do right by people. I may be sick and in a lot of pain, but I have peace that you can't even imagine.

Since I was a teenager, I had been in a sexual relationship with either a boyfriend or a husband. These last nine years and counting, not having sex has been the most liberating period of my life. Now I know many people say they can't go that long without sex. Believe me, I didn't think I could go that long without sex. My marriage made sex so ugly and illicit. All I could picture in my head was all these people--

anyone and everyone he could convince to have sex with him; it made me never want to have sex again.

I wish I could say I first decided to stop having sex because I wanted to be faithful to God. But I stopped because the thought of it with him was YUCK! And the result has become a commitment to do what's right in the sight of God. I am not perfect. I'm just trying to do what's right and do right by people.

I have this calculation that I used in a sermon and in lessons I have taught in teen sessions. Let's use for example that John met Joan, and they lie together. That's 2 people. But John previously slept with 5 other individuals before he met Joan. So now we are at 7. But Joan slept with 5 other individuals before she met John, so now we are at 12. But each of those 10 individuals, (5 for John and 5 for Joan) also slept with 5 individuals before John met Joan. So that's 50 other people. So just with this one sexual encounter, you could possibly be picking up something from 62 people. This is just one example to give us something to think about.

It's funny the things that shape your course in life. The day my husband spoke these words to me, "I married beneath me," I knew in my heart my life as I knew it was over. As devastating as those words were when they hit my heart, they also were so empowering. The strength I needed to change our situation and the ability to clearly see what my life had become came into clear focus. I knew no matter how low or beneath anyone felt that I was to them, God saw something more. The word says God will bring back to your remembrance his word. And what came back to my mind was you are "above" and not "beneath."

When others look at you as nothing, God sees something. God sees the part of you that He finds worthy to save, restore, and redeem. I knew I deserved more. I knew I deserved to spend my last days in the presence of people who loved me and thought more highly of me. I knew I could no longer spend another second with someone who could speak words as if they despised me. We all deserve to surround ourselves with love and peace. We also all deserve to spend our moments with someone who sees worth in your relationship and to spend our days knowing we are loved, and the love we give in turn is reciprocated.

I had to ask the question, "Why have I purposely chosen to spend my days unappreciated and looked at as worthless?" God has more. And all of us deserve more. We deserve to live our lives to the full capacity that God has ordained for us in our lives. Our God has promised us abundantly more than we could ask or think. Our God has come that we may have life and have it more abundantly.

Dear friends, if you are feeling unloved know that God loves you unconditionally. He loves you like no other can. He can deposit in you a love and forgiveness like never before that will show to all the people you meet. If there is nothing to hold on to, hold on to God's love.

So who am I? I pray that I can be found only as a humble servant of our mighty God.

Chapter 11
One of Those Days

This is not a good day. The spasms in my neck, shoulders, and back are sending pain through me like you wouldn't believe. This is the forth straight day of continuous pain. At this moment I am fully medicated with everything I have in this house that I could possibly take. The microwave heating pad is planted around my neck. God has blessed me with the most wonderful friends. My Deaconess learned that I was having pain in my neck, so she came over with all her potions and remedies. She massaged my neck and gave me this stuff that really worked. She is one of those people who God sent to me directly from heaven. The moment she found out I was HIV positive, she and her husband have gone out of their way to help me in any way they can. They have been close friends for years. They have suffered through everything my family has suffered, right alongside us.

After my husband trashed our house and cut up all my furniture, they were the first ones there to help me clean up. Her husband, my wonderful Pastor, who has since passed away, and our Trustee came to my house. They cleaned all the trash out of the house and helped me get it into some kind of shape to sell it. Of course, the mortgage company made sure I did not receive anything from the sale of the house, but I was just glad the house was sold.

These are the kinds of people God has blessed me with. My prayer is that many people will find church members who will rally around them with nothing but love and support. Isn't this how it should be? If we can't confide in our own church family and not receive rejection, then who can we confide in? Okay, this pain will not let me sit at this computer today; it's taking over my thoughts, and I can no longer concentrate. Doctors keep telling me I shouldn't still be having this much pain from the accident. Will somebody please tell that to my neck!

Chapter 12

No, I Didn't End Up in Another Crazy Emergency Room

I could not make this stuff up if I wanted to. You will not believe what has happened to me again. I think these hospitals are trying to force me to march around their emergency rooms with picket signs.

It was 3:00 a.m. in the morning. My heart was racing so fast, and it felt like it was going to jump out of my chest. I was being squeezed around my chest, and it hurt so bad I could not think. It felt like I had on a really tight bra, but I didn't have one on. I woke up my daughter, and she called the ambulance. I am laid out on the couch. This man comes into my house, moving slower than a snail. He's checking my pressure and heart, and says he thinks it is okay, but I can go to the emergency room if I want to. IF I WANT TO--ARE YOU KIDDING ME? Now while he's checking me out, he is also singing, and humming. I am not saying a word, unless he asks me a question.

Finally they take me to this crazy hospital in the Germantown section of Philadelphia, Pennsylvania. Let it be known now and forever more--don't ever take me to that crazy hospital again as long as I live! My daughter followed in the ambulance. She has my purse with my medication list and insurance cards. The nurse takes me into the intake room. I have told her that I am having chest pains, and I have to go to the bathroom. I also informed her that my daughter should be right behind us with the list. She totally ignores me as if I have not said a word. She makes me sit up in this chair for over 30 minutes. CHEST PAIN is NOT a concern of HERS! Please note the CHEST PAIN is a BIG concern of MINE!!

She asked what medicine I took. I have a list of over 18 medications. I say again, "My daughter is right behind us. She has the list in my purse." She again asks, "I need to know your medications." I asked if we could please call my daughter because she has the list. "Just tell me the medications," she demanded. I tried to name all that I can remember. As soon as I mentioned the HIV drugs, her entire demeanor gets even worse, if you think that could be possible. The look of disgust went to her face. She is just typing on the computer. I am in this chair feeling like I am going to pass out and pee on myself at the same time. She is totally ignoring me and just typing. I ask again for my daughter. She tells me no, she can't call my daughter. I have to get the medications in the computer first. I plead again if we could please get my daughter she has my information. She refused to get my daughter. After 30 minutes, she then places me in a room and begins to get my vital signs. She leaves me there for another 40 minutes, coming in the room every now and then. I am begging to go to the bathroom and for my daughter. She completely ignores me.

Finally she hooks me up to an EKG machine. She determines that my heartbeat is not normal, and now rushes to call the doctor. The doctor comes in and is very courteous. I tell her that I need to go to the bathroom really badly, and that my daughter followed the ambulance in the car. The doctor has the nurse get me a bedpan, and then tries to find my daughter. I hear them in the hall saying my daughter wants to come back. The nurse tells them that she can't come back because I am on the bedpan. She left me on that bedpan for another 30 minutes. The doctor finally comes back and takes me off the bedpan. I tell her I hear my daughter's name, and she allows my daughter to finally come back.

I learn from my daughter that she was in the waiting room the entire time. She has been begging to come back, but they kept telling her the nurse said she could not come back. I could not believe it. They put this patch of nitro on my chest for my heart. This slows up my heart rate. It felt like it feels when my sugar drops low. I am telling my daughter to call the nurse. Now a male nurse is on duty, and he tells her I have to wait. She tells him again something is wrong. He won't come in the room. Another person who was not assigned to me saw on the monitor that my heart rate had dropped, and she rushed in the room to help me and called the doctor. The doctor is trying to help, and the male nurse comes up to me and tells me to stop breathing like that. I don't know what he is talking about; all I can remember is trying to catch my breath. I am afraid that these people might kill me. He is holding on to me then just lets me go. My body just dropped in the bed.

I am crying, and my daughter is now crying. She cannot believe how these people are treating me. She calls my family. By now it is morning. They are telling me that I have to be transferred to another hospital because of my heart. I tell them I want to go to my hospital where my primary doctor is located. After the doctors called back and forth on the phone, they tell me they cannot take me to my hospital. But my family is in agreement--they have to get me out of here because we don't know how I will end up if left in the hands of these rude and clearly uncaring people who are treating me as if I am not worthy of their concern.

My family places me in a wheelchair and tells them to give us the discharge papers because we are leaving. They tell us they're busy and don't have time to do the papers, I'll have to wait. We had enough. They immediately wheeled me right out of that hospital. Now the people are saying you can't take her until you sign these papers. She hollers back, OH, now you have time to prepare the papers. They took me out of there and straight to my hospital which is Presbyterian Hospital. I don't care what anyone says about this hospital because they have treated me with more love and kindness than any other emergency room I have been in. I have the most wonderful doctors in the world. So for all of you in Philadelphia looking for caring, compassionate doctors, I've found the best--Dr. Griska, Dr. Silverman and Dr. Vigilante.

If I am too sick and not able to speak for myself, please take me to any of these three doctors.

I pray some hospital administrator reads this and uses it as a guide to train their staff on how not to treat patients. If I may please offer a suggestion, treat patients like you're treating your own mother.

Chapter 13

Why Write?

Why write and why share all of my personal information? I am a lone voice in a silent issue. I am writing this book in hopes of helping those who are suffering alone. I write to all who have this disease and to all who may know someone with this disease. And I write to all who may face this disease in the future. To all who may want to know what it feels like to have this disease. And most importantly to anyone who has wrongly treated any individual just because they have this disease. To them I can only say be careful. In this lifetime you truly do reap what you sow. I wanted to share this experience and say things that many people would love to say, but are scared; they are scared that they may be shunned, treated differently, or may be ousted from their families.

If you are suffering, I want you to know that you are not alone. God Loves You. I love you, and as long as I am on this earth, I am here to suffer along with you--to share in your joys and sorrows. You may not believe what I believe, but pain knows no religion, pain knows no race, pain knows no gender. But pain does know our name. This disease has affected people from every walk of life. I know many do not believe in what I believe. I know many have chosen alternative lifestyles. But no matter what choices we've made-- good or bad--God loves us unconditionally. *"God so loved the world, that he gave his only begotten son, that whosoever, believeth in him should not perish, but have everlasting life." (John 3:16 kjv)*

Therefore, whoever you are and whatever you have done, I must love you unconditionally. His forgiveness is never ending, and our forgiveness should be never ending. Forgiveness is a powerful tool. I have begun to pray daily for my enemies. I have begun to pray blessings on their lives and families. I pray for their prosperity, hopes, dreams, and abundant blessings to fall upon them. I pray for a release for all the wrongs perceived and actual. I pray that God releases me from all anger, hatred, and bitterness so that those same feelings they have toward me may also be released.

You cannot believe the release I felt in my heart once I began to do this. I literally felt better, and joy leapt in my soul. A smile came to my face, and a peace you would not believe. I began to see them in my mind prospering and it made me happy. My eyes were opened and the true sense of forgiveness that had previously evaded me was now mine. I wasn't always at this point. God had to bring me to this point.

I'll share later the story of my praying for a good friend and how the sense of urgency and pleading to God for her deliverance brought me to tears. In the midst of my prayer, God's convicting power was so present that it scared me. I crumbled in tears asking for God's forgiveness. I've been sincerely praying for my enemies, my ex-husband, and anyone who has hurt me ever since. The freedom of Forgiveness is a wonderful tool. Use daily.

(Psalm 66:18 kjv) "If I regard iniquity in my heart, the Lord will not hear me."

Chapter 14
My Year of Jubilee

Some may think, "How can you call this your year of Jubilee? You lost your brother, then your mother. Your apartment was flooded, and you lost almost all of its contents. And the few things that remain are sitting right next to you, piled up in heavy duty trash bags in the area where a completely furnished living room set once occupied. How can you say this is your year to celebrate?" Things are not always what they seem. I can truly declare this statement from the core of my being. When life gives you downs, look for the ups! This year God fulfilled promises in my life that I thought I would not live to see. I saw the age of 50 on November 15, 2009! You could not have told me in 1991 that I would live to see age 50. I shouted for JOY on my 50th birth date. My daughters surprised me with a birthday party. Then they showed a video they prepared of our beautiful life, and what I meant to them and my family. They had pictures of my entire family, and messages of love from each of them. It was the most moving thing I had ever seen. There was not a dry eye in the room. I will treasure that video for the remainder of my life. The video has been posted to YouTube so you can watch it too. The link is: http://youtu.be/5ymZkK_cImk

My experience always reminds me of the blind man that Jesus healed. The Pharisees wanted this man to accuse Jesus, but his response was, *"Whether he be a sinner or no, I know not. One thing I know that whereas I was blind, now I see." (John 9:25 kjv)*

One thing I know to be true is over six years ago, God spoke a prophetic word into my life to let me know that I will live to see my girls graduate. I was suffering from severe depression, and did not know it. The enemy had me convinced that I would die from HIV/AIDS before these children would grow up. At a conference, I heard a sermon by a well spoken and wonderful man of God. He wove into his sermon the story of an unbeatable chess match. After careful examination of the match by a chess master, he declared it was a lie; the match was beatable. The word our Lord and Master gave me that night was, "It's a lie; you will live and not die."

I left that conference on a spiritual high. I felt in my spirit that things were going to change at that moment. But I have learned that God's time is not our time. When things did not change when I expected them to change, I let go of that promise. I did not remember this promise when suffering through some of the hardest moments in my life. I remained bound for years after the promise.

Here now, in my year of Jubilee, one thing I know is that whereas I was bound, now I am free. I declared in 2012 that I have lived 22 years with HIV. In the year 2012, my 5-year-old is now 27, and with these eyes, I saw her graduate from Delaware State University. Whereas that 9-month-old baby is now 22, and with these eyes I saw her graduate from high school with honors, and with these hands, I moved her into Temple University. With these feet, I walked to the polls with young women, whom God blessed me to see live, and we voted as a family. I just walked down the street behind them with a smile on my face, as I praised God on the inside. Only God could have brought me to this point. I kept taking pictures, they of course were like, "Mom why are you so hyped?" If I could bottle that feeling and they could taste it, they would understand. *"Taste and see that the Lord is good." (Psalm 34:8 kjv)* I am alive. I am living to see exceedingly, abundantly more than I could ask or think. I am just walking down the street, but I am celebrating. All I can say is you have to live it.

God truly has given me abundantly more than I could ask or think. One thing I know to be true is that a prophetic word, spoken by a profound man of God, was spoken into my life. Once I was bound, but now I'm Free. *"So if the Son sets you free, you will be free indeed." (John 8:36 kjv)*

I've had some downs this year, but the ups have immensely outweighed the downs. I rejoice in these tribulations because I see all things working together for my good. I shout through every trial because I now look at them all as an opportunity to minister to someone else who I may meet in need. If I am going through it, then I am going to meet someone who needs a word of encouragement who has gone through the same thing.

I see now that I needed to suffer through depression as a result of being diagnosed with HIV. When I meet someone who is newly diagnosed, I know exactly where they are at spiritually and mentally. I immediately begin to pray, and ask God to give me a word that will inspire them and lift them up. And time and time again, he gives me a word, directly from my experiences, to speak life into their situation. This year I have become thankful for being able to share and talk with others suffering from this disease.

For 12 years of my marriage, I had no one to talk with concerning HIV. When I give it a lot of thought, I had no one to talk to concerning many of the fears and deep issues I needed to discuss. I was scared to talk with my family. I did not want to make them sad and depressed, so I just talked about happy times and happy things. Anything real stayed inside. It wasn't until I began to see a therapist that I began to open up.

My husband never wanted to discuss it. He did not want to hear the word. The moment I would get HIV out of my mouth, I'd be shut down with, "I don't want to talk about it now." Speaking is my chance to talk, release and pour out all I have been holding in for a long time. With each word I feel freed from the pain. With each word, I am finding understanding and clarity. And the amazing part is that as I am releasing everything and pouring out my soul, forgiveness is being released into the atmosphere.

When I see others being encouraged by my story and given the strength to seek the help and guidance they need, I see God's purpose being fulfilled in my life. Chapters of my life are closing, and there are so many new beginnings. I am not bound. I am not locked up. Writing is like freedom. Talking is freedom. All I can say is, "If the Son set you free, you will be free indeed."

In January of this year, God called my brother Herman "Smitty" Smith home to his eternal rest in Glory. My entire family misses him so much. His leaving us brought back so many memories of when my sister Carolyn King died in 1998. The two siblings who were full of so much life were gone. I love focusing on how much fun they were. Carol traveled all over this country. But when she came home, it was like a party. There's so many of us, it was always like a party, but when Carol was home, it was time to celebrate.

Mom cooked all her favorite foods. We enjoyed every minute of her, until it was time for her to leave town. Smitty we loved to tease because he knew everyone, everywhere. You could not go anywhere with him, without him hollering out the car window saying "hey" to every person walking down the street. I would always say, "Smitty, you don't know them." He would say, "Yes I do, Di," and then proceed to tell me their life story. But I can celebrate them even in death, because I know I loved them every moment I could while they were here. No one knows the day or hour when God will call you home. I know I have repeated this several times, but I am so grateful for every second. For so many years I was convinced that I would be leaving this earth before any of my brothers and sisters. God's plan is not our plan. So count your blessings for the lives that are all around you. I want to live my life as God has instructed, so that when I leave this earth, I will spend an eternity in the same place as my sister, brother, and my mother. You may have family suffering from this disease. Maybe because of their lifestyle, you cannot let them in. Find it in your heart to let them in before it is too late. Love them while you have a chance. Give them the love that you would hope to receive.

Our heavenly father called our Mother home September 16, 2008. This happening at any other time in my life may have sent me into deeper depression. But I rejoice because of what God blessed my mother and me with that year. My Mom was crazy about all of her grandchildren. She poured into these children all the love any person could humanly give. My mom was so excited that my daughters and my niece were graduating that year. She was there for all three graduations and all three parties. One of the nicest last pictures of my mom and dad was taken at my niece's party.

My mom's last visit was a surprise for my daughter and niece's college send-off parties. I prayed when these children were 5 years old and 9 months old that God would bless me to live to see my children graduate. And in 2008 God granted my request. But he granted me abundantly more than I could ask when he allowed my Mom to live to experience these wonderful achievements. It was almost like she prayed to see this as well, and then God called her home. I prayed that I would live to see them graduate from high school. God blessed my mom and me to see my oldest daughter graduate from college and the youngest graduate from high school. My youngest daughter got accepted into every college she applied to except for one. We saw her move into her dorm, and I can only thank God.

As I said earlier, no one knows the day or hour when God will call you home. Make every moment count. I did not realize how much my mom worried about my death until God called her home. We began to go through her papers and found all the mementos that she had been preparing for my death. All the precious memories she was storing up for my children. She had pictures of me put aside to use on the obituary. She wrote a poem to be included in my obituary. She had messages for the children. She was preparing to lose a daughter. Because she thought she would lose a daughter, she gave all the love and support a parent could give while she had a chance.

I'm trying to write and share with you this experience, but it is hard through the tears. This disease does not just ravage you mentally and spiritually, but it wasn't until I read all my mom's notes that I realized just how much my diagnosis was on her mind. She worried about me daily. She worried about the future of my children daily. Just as I have spent the past 22 years dealing with this disease, my mom and families all around the world are suffering along with the victims of this disease.

It affects our entire family in ways we can't even begin to imagine. They may not share it with you, but it consumes all of us. If I had known she was this worried about me, I would have talked to her more about it. But I always felt no one wanted to keep talking about AIDS because it was such a downer. Now I am filled with such sadness that this may have had my mom down for years. When I was suffering, she was suffering. Whatever is happening to our children is happening to us.

I recently preached a sermon from (Matthew 15:25-27 kjv): *"The woman came and knelt before him. 'Lord, help me!' she said. 26He replied, 'It is not right to take the children's bread and toss it to their dogs.' 27'Yes, Lord,' she said, 'but even the dogs eat the crumbs that fall from their masters' table.'"* This mother came to Christ for her sick child. But in verse 25 she yells, *"Lord, Help ME!"* This statement screams: my daughter is suffering, therefore I'm suffering. And her cry was for herself. But here faith knew if He helped her, it would transfer to her household.

I would love a chance to talk with my mom about all the wonderful things she wrote in her letters and notes. I know my mom is gone, but I keep thinking of all these things I want to say to her. I'm telling myself I have to tell mom that. Then I fill with such sadness because I can't. It hurts when I think of all the signs I missed.

Several weeks before my mom passed, I had a dream of Herman in a coffin. In this dream I thought it was my brother; but I said to myself when I woke up,

"Herman looked like Mom with a fatter face." When my mom passed and her face was much fatter from all the fluids, her face was exactly as I saw her in my dreams. As we were about to leave the house to head for the hospital on the day before my mom passed, my dad was telling my daughter and me how Mom thinks she is in our old house on Pemberton Street where we lived for over 30 something years. I always heard stories of people saying loved ones believed they saw people and places from years prior. When I left the hospital the night before her heart stopped, as I was walking down the hall, something said, "Go back." But I kept telling myself, she has the tube going through her nose, she's shivering, and I don't want her to talk; I just want to let her rest. So I won't bother her anymore tonight. I'll just be here first thing in the morning. Being able to speak again never came for her in the morning. I did not get that morning. That morning was not promised. What I would give at this moment for an opportunity to turn around and go back. I'm sorry, I can't stop crying, and the screen is blurry through all my tears. This is all I am going to be able to write about my mom.

You may be preparing to leave this earth because you've received a medical diagnosis that may not be very promising. But I say don't wait for a diagnosis to make every moment count. Make every moment count because you have been given a gift of precious time--a gift that if wasted, cannot be returned.

Chapter 15

A Sermon Worth Sharing

I am moved today to share a sermon that I wrote for a speaking engagement to talk about my experience with HIV. I thank God for the invitation. I have been invited to speak at a lot of places, but this is the first time I was asked to deliver a sermon specifically pertaining to HIV. My goal for sharing this sermon in this book is a hope that someone suffering with the isolation of HIV may be encouraged.

Sermon Title: Yet Will I Trust HIM

My reason for being here today is simple. God has brought me to it, so he will bring me through it. And He has brought me through it to help others. Time and time again He has showed His awesome wonder, His awesome power, and His awesome grace.

"All things work together for the good, for those that Love the Lord and are the called according to his purpose." (Romans 8:28 kjv)

How is HIV working together for my good? Well hindsight is 20/20. You will see by the time we are done, how it has worked for my good. But the purpose in which he has me here today is Love. Can I love them, in spite of? Can I forgive them, in spite of? Can I live, in spite of? And the word for us today is, yes we can.

Because if we ever want a change to occur in our lives, we first have to examine some of the areas that God requires some things from us.

There is always a scripture that can be applied to any situation we encounter in life. And there is a word from the Lord which I believe will be very beneficial for each of us as we strive to help those living with AIDS and HIV--and that word truly is LOVE.

*"A new command I give you: **Love one another**. As I have **loved** you, so you must **love one another**. By this all men will know that you are my disciples, if you **love one another**."* That scripture comes from (John 13:34 & 35 kjv).

I'd like you to keep the word LOVE in mind as we go through our discussions, and I'd like us to just think about the thought, "What if God were to pick and choose whom He was going to save instead of His willingness to save the entire world?" Aren't you glad that he wants to save everybody? Because I'm thinking with some of the mess I've done, I might not have made it through the screening process. If all the drug addicts, fornicators, and gossipers weren't allowed in, I wouldn't have made the cut. If truth be told, some of you might not have made the cut either. But He said, *"Who so ever will, come."* (Mark 8:34 kjv) Aren't you glad about it?

How did it become okay to shun people living with HIV/AIDS? How did it become okay to treat people negatively based on the way they contracted this disease? When did it become okay to hate people because of their sexual orientation?

I have had some very interesting encounters as a result of people finding out I am HIV positive. The blessing for me is that I have a wonderful supportive family, a wonderful church family, and a great group of friends. But there are a lot of people suffering, dying, and living in loneliness and isolation because of this disease. My prayer is that today we will leave here with enough Love in our Hearts that we can:

"Love everyone in spite of,

In spite of what I look like,

In spite of what I've done,

In spite of my sins,

And don't get it twisted and think I am singling out the sins of any particular group, as hard as it is. Sometimes you have to look within and accept the reality that all have sinned and fallen short of the glory of God." (Rom. 3:23 kjv)

Seems like if there are some folks in need of love, there ought to be something we can pull from the many things we have learned about how to treat one another. Maybe some parable we could pull out of a hat that may be beneficial for such a time as this.

Let's take the parable of the Good Samaritan. The Jews didn't have dealings with the Samaritans. A Jew lies robbed and beaten on the side of the road. A Priest sees him, crosses to the other side, and passes him by. A Levite sees him and crosses to the other side and passes him by. But the Samaritan had pity on him. He picked him up, fixed his wounds, took him to an inn, took care of him, and left money for him to be able to stay at the inn. His own people refused to touch him.

Let's go pick our sisters and brothers up from the side of the road and show them some love. Their side of the road could be lying in a dark bedroom suffering with depression. (Been there done that.) Their side of the road might be standing on a street corner, giving away their body because they feel unworthy. (Let's go pick 'em up from the side of the road.) They may be sad and lonely because they've contracted a disease, and no one wants to touch them anymore. (Let's go pick 'em up from the side of the road.)

In this parable, Jesus said the neighbor was, *"He that shewed mercy on him." (Luke 10:37)* His instruction to them was, *"Go, and do thou likewise." (Luke 10:37)* What can we do? Search for a way to meet people where they are and show them unconditional love.

What does God require from us for our brethren who have fallen into diverse temptations? He wants us to go and pick them up from the side of the road.

I have to speak out because of what God has done in my life. Some may look at my life and see heartache, pain, failure, misery. This is exactly how I saw it at one point. But today I see promise, purpose, meaning, hope, joy, and all things working together for my Good. So I have to do what I can in hopes that someone else may be pulled from their dark place into His marvelous light.

I have two lists. They represent the way I saw everything that has happened to me, and the way I now see everything that has happened to me.

This list represents how I used to see my life:

- I found out I was HIV positive. I have a five-year-old and 9-month-old baby
- I suffered from years of depression
- I went back on drugs
- I tried to kill myself via self destruction
- I settled for this relationship
- My husband had a baby by another woman on my 1st wedding anniversary
- My sister died
- I suffered through years of arguments and verbal abuse
- I found out my husband spent all our money on drugs and prostitutes
- Our church fell apart
- My husband kicked me in my stomach
- He told me, "I married beneath me."

- He refused to leave our home
- I had to flee my home
- My husband destroyed my belongings and our home
- The house went into foreclosure, and I was left with all the bills
- We had to move in with my mom and dad
- There was barely any room for us
- I got sick and ended up in the hospital
- I was in physical therapy
- A kid slammed into the back of my car, and in addition to all the other problems, I now have herniated discs in my neck and back
- Now I am back in physical therapy
- I still get spasms in my neck and back
- I can't work
- I lost my job during my daughter's first year of college
- I was hospitalized with fever and infection. They found out my kidneys are failing, I had an irregular

heartbeat, and I am at risk for heart disease. My lung capacity is reduced. I needed two pints of blood. I now have to take insulin for my diabetes

- I lost my medical insurance
- After a 30-year work history, I am now on welfare
- I am repeatedly denied social security
- My car gives out
- My brother died
- Our apartment is flooded
- We lost all our furniture and most of mine and the children's clothes
- Then I lost my mom

That's one way of looking at my life. But here is how God has worked all that out for my good. And here is my new way of looking at my life:

- Because of this disease, I begin to value time. No one knows the day or hour, so I decide that every second I get with my kids is going to count.
- I dedicate my life to Christ.
- I completely gave up all drugs.

- I joined a wonderful church and get to help some wonderful children.
- I told my sister about the goodness of Christ before she passed.
- When our church fell apart, we received a wonderful Pastor, Joseph Hutchinson and his lovely wife Viveca. He preached forgiveness and healing to our congregation, and God's words truly ministered to me during this period.
- All the women of the church surrounded me with their love and would not let me go.
- Pastor Hutchinson, Deacon Phillips, and Minister Nate rented a dumpster and cleaned out my house so I could sell it and not have a foreclosure on my record.
- I had a mom and dad who were more than willing to take my family in.
- I was able to get medical assistance and get the treatment and medication I needed.
- I was finally approved for social security.
- With the back payments, we were able to catch up on our bills and keep my daughter in college.

- They caught my kidney disease before I had to go on dialysis.
- I received an apartment without a dime.
- After sitting in utter agony in church, I was experiencing worship like never before.
- Pastor Hutchinson signed me up for Ministerial Training.
- My teacher was Pastor André Seals. When God called Pastor Hutchinson home, my teacher became my Pastor. He encouraged me to continue training.
- We lost a car, but my daughter still has her car.
- I prayed to live to see my daughters graduate from high school.
- My oldest not only graduated from high school but also graduated from Delaware State.
- My youngest graduated from high school with honors, was accepted to just about every college she applied, and is now at Temple University.
- My mom lived long enough to see all this happen, and it brought her immense joy.

- God has taken my CD 4 count from the 200's to the 700's, and my viral load from the 6,000's to "zero". In other words "undetectable"!
- I shared the good news of Jesus Christ with my brother before he died, and he accepted Christ as his personal Savior.
- God brought me to North Carolina to have a chance to see my mom before she passed.

You can spend your life focusing on the downs, but I am going to focus on the ups. Ball up every bad issue that has happened in your life and cast them into the pits of hell, and then speak into existence every good and perfect gift that has come from above.

I am the head and not the tail.

I am above and not beneath.

He whom the Son sets free is free indeed.

You are a chosen people.

A royal priesthood.

A holy nation.

A people belonging to God.

He called me out of darkness into His marvelous light.

I have never seen the righteous forsaken nor His seed begging bread.

He will do exceedingly, abundantly more than I can ask or think

I will praise Thee, for I am fearfully and wonderfully made; marvelous are Thy works, and that my soul knoweth right well.

Think on those things that are kind; think on those things that are pure; think on those things that are just.

I could focus on that list of negative thoughts.

But I choose to focus on the positive ones.

In this list I see all things working together for my good.

In this list I see a purpose and plans being revealed.

In this list I see reasons to get up.

Tell someone you love to get a good list and hold on to that.

Before we open up the floor for questions, there is one more area that I believe is very important to share.

I haven't had sex since about three months before I left my husband in 2003. And it's not because I am so holy or that in the beginning I was doing this for God.

No, if truth be told, I did not set out to be obedient in this area. The problem was that I was so turned off because of all the visuals I had in my head of all these people sleeping in my house and in my bed every day as soon as I left for work. I worked the day shift, and he worked the night shift. And I just kept thinking about all these spirits that entered my body every time I lay down with him. And if you don't know, spirits are transferred through sex and laying on of hands.

Now let me just add a side bar. Folks, we are going to have to get better at helping a sister out. After I left my husband, my neighbor then told me all the horror stories of all the people who were going in and out of my house while I was at work. She could have given a sister a heads-up. I know some people don't want to know. But as for me, I really want to know.

It did not start as a faith thing, but through it, God has allowed me to experience some wonderful blessings by putting sexual things under check.

Don't get me wrong, I could rumble with the best of them, but that's flesh.

And if truth be told, our flesh has already gotten us in this situation and many other pretty bad situations. But when you can bring that flesh under control, no, let me rephrase: If you can allow God to help you bring your flesh under control, tell Him, "I am weak, and I need you to help me in this area." Trust me, you'll be glad you did.

So I received an unexpected blessing in this area. I began to notice when I would get my blood work, my numbers began to rise. I really hadn't given it much thought, but before I knew it, 6 years had passed and my T cell counts went from the 200's up to 700's, and the viral load count went from 6,000's to undetectable.

I had unknowingly kept my body as a living sacrifice, and in being obedient in this area, God had blessed me with counts that I didn't know I was able to achieve again. I thought once they went down, I was destined for them to stay down. But I am my own scientific proof that you can reverse this thing by just not allowing yourself to be re-infected over and over again every time you sleep with someone who is infected. And you must also be taking your medication every day.

I started thinking about that scripture, *"If my people, which are called by my name, shall humble themselves, and pray, and seek my face, and turn from their wicked ways; then will I hear from heaven, and will forgive their sin, and will heal their land."* (II Chronicles 7:14 kjv) So I started telling myself that I am people in the land, and if you're going to heal the land, then you have to heal the people in the land, so I'm willing to humble myself, turn from my wicked ways, strive for obedience, and continue to look for my healing.

I'll be the first one to tell you that if there is ever a day and time to be abstinent, that day and time would be now. But the reality is that everyone is not going to stop having sex, so I will also be the first one to tell you to use a condom. Don't suffer like I have. This illness is no joke. This disease is spreading rapidly through our communities, and unfortunately the teen population is becoming one of the highest populations being infected.

I can put myself out here because I am just so happy that Jesus saved me from my mess that I just want to serve him in any capacity that I can. And if sharing my story will help one person to not have to suffer like I have, then I'll do it. I promised Him, "Here am I Lord, send me."

So I pray that I have been obedient in doing what he has called me to do. Thank you for having me here today, and thank you for allowing me to share. God Bless You.

Chapter 16

Why Are There So Many Questions After Death?

Is it normal to still have so many questions when a person has passed away? My ex-husband has passed away. And yet, I still have so many questions that remain unanswered. We talked many times after the years we separated and then later divorced. But whenever the subject went to the various scenarios we encountered over the years, we immediately had to change the subject because we could see an argument was about to occur. I would have to say, "I'm sorry I can't argue anymore. My arguing days are over."

I don't want to have to ever argue again. So the topics stayed safe. How are the kids? How are your parents? I can't find this or that paper. Have you seen it, etc.? I always told him about my speaking engagements and how open I am about our lives as well as everything that had happened. He said he was happy that I was able to talk, but he wasn't ready to talk about it. I shared the freedom of writing and talking.

As preachers of the gospel, we have been entrusted to tell others the good news of the love of Jesus Christ and how He has come to give them life and a more abundant life. But I found myself in a marriage where my husband was telling others the things of God that he believed he was instructed to tell them. But there was an entirely different life hidden from his wife. While others were being told the good news, there were a few things I should have been told. Today, although it's too late, I still ask: What had God told you to tell your wife? What were the hidden truths of your heart? What are the things the Pastor never told his wife? We were sent to tell others so much, but the truth of ourselves stayed hidden. All I have left is my own truth and that is Love hurts. Love lifts. Love inspires. Love learns how to let go when it's not reciprocated. Every act of betrayal burned to the core. But every act is being used today to tell someone you can and will recover from the worst pain ever. God can and will lift you from that pain and bring you to a place of peace where you can completely rest in Him and the power of his forgiveness. He'll give you the strength to share your worst pain ever, and the power to encourage others. I don't know what this wife wasn't told, but I want to tell you every word God gives me that can bring you from your place of hurt.

I want to give you words that will bring you from your place of fear, your place of loneliness, your place of darkness, and that instead will take you to a place of love in the arms of a God that loves you unconditionally. In spite of what you have endured, you can be made whole. We have to ask ourselves, do we want to be made whole, or do we want to stay in that pain we cannot change? I wanted to be made whole.

The conversation I am most thankful for is the, "I forgive you conversation." Early after the separation and a counseling session, he called and I told him I forgave him. He also said he forgave me. But I am more thankful for the second "I forgive you conversation" we were able to have.

A dear friend of mine was going through some trouble. I went to visit her and just sat outside on the steps and poured out all my mistakes, drug use, and depression and how God delivered me from them. As soon as I arrived home, I went into prayer for her. My heart was so broken for her. I loved her and went into earnest prayer for her deliverance. I began to cry out to the Lord on her behalf. The tears were streaming down my face. And right in the midst of this prayer, I heard the Lord say as clear as day, "Can you cry out to me for the soul of your ex-husband? Can you shed tears for his deliverance?" I was so convicted. I believed I forgave him. But I had not shed tears for him. I had shed bottles full of tears. Those shed tears were for me, my own hurt, and my own pain.

That day I apologized to God and shed tears for him. God required a sincere forgiveness. He required unconditional love. That did not mean allow yourself to be abused and taken advantage of, but love him as God has loved me. Release every pain and hurt into God's hands. I will handle your pain and hurt, but he is now in need of someone who loves him to go into earnest, tearful, heartfelt prayer. Are you willing?

That day I prayed for his soul. I prayed for his deliverance. I prayed that he would feel God's Love for him encamped around him. That day I shed tears for his soul. And the next time he called, I told him the story and I told him I forgave him, and I knew it was sincere. I knew God had allowed me to let go. I could tell that he knew it was sincere.

Even today, I know it's too late, but I have so many questions. The root of all this destruction was sex. Sex took my health, my home, my marriage, my job, and my finances. Was it worth it? I'm sorry, I've had a whole lot of sex in my lifetime, and I have never come across any that was so good that I was willing to give up all that I had for the experience. But that is what was allowed to happen.

I know he is no longer with us, but that question won't leave my head, was it worth it?

Maybe it won't leave my head because someone may read this that is about to let sex destroy his or her life, and they need to ask the question: "Is this really worth it?"

I want to know did he apologize to those women? Did he tell them to get tested? I want to find them and tell them to get tested. I want to tell them I'm not mad at them. Just get yourself tested. I want to stop the spread. I pray for the women who may not know that God will make a way for them to get tested.

I question what could have been. Why do we long, even when it is over, for what could have been? What if there was complete trust and faithfulness. What if we always took our medicine and took care of our bodies, would he still be here? I know it doesn't matter now, but I even question was I truly loved. After all these years, I still don't know the answer to that question, and I have to accept the fact that I never will. But my solace and the answer to that question is what really matters for us all and that is Jesus Christ loves us unconditionally. And that's enough.

But this morning I have come as close as I believe I will to answering some of my questions. I sit and write early this morning. I have just awoken from a dream of the perfect date with my ex-husband. He is still my husband in this dream. We are on one of our many getaways. We are at the perfect hotel. It's cozy, warm, and full of other couples retreating away to alone time. We check and double check our bags for our medications and all the essentials we may need for our trip. We awaken with coffee and conversation-- our daily routine. Our medication is set on the table. I am making sure that he hasn't forgotten anything, and he reassures me that I haven't forgotten anything. We eat a wonderful breakfast, take our medication, and begin to plan the perfect day.

Our day would consist of dinner and a movie. We begin to dress. It's one of the rare moments that I am not wearing a wig. He never liked my wigs and today I am wearing my hair in a perfect style, and I am having a great hair day. He comments on how pretty my hair looks, and thanks me for having it done for him. I check his outfit, and he checks mine. We both agree that we look very nice. I proceed to put on my make-up. I receive a phone call and immediately say, "I can't talk right now. I'm getting dressed for a date, but if you're still awake, I can call you in a couple of hours." My date came first. I was willing to put everything else aside. This was a special moment. Everything else had to wait.

Then my perfect date began to fall apart. While I tried to put on my make-up, people were trying to get into the bathroom. I was then being rushed to a car. The car we were driving in was not our car. I asked where the car came from. He said it wasn't ours, so we have to hurry because someone is after us. Then I awoke. I awoke and realized that someone was after us for over 32 years. Someone, God, life was trying to lead us in perfect harmony, and we never grasped it. We did not get it. What is IT? Two people who desire to become the one that God has ordained from the beginning of time. Two people in sync. Two people willing to put the cares of life on hold and take time out for the perfect date.

I desired a marriage that did not exist in my household. We allowed anything and everything to come first. We placed everything before what was most important. I'll never get my questions answered any more than I'll be able to reverse anything that has taken place. So where do you go from here? You learn. You learn that sometimes you don't get a second chance. If you have something of value, then value it while it is in your grasp. Don't take it for granted. Don't believe it will always be there. Realize that some things are not meant to be. Your priorities may not be another individual's priorities. What they desire in life may not be what you desire in life. Know when it's time to let go. Know when it is time to hold on. Know when it's time for a new dream.

Chapter 17

Lessons Learned As
We Head for the Inevitable

In the end, there is only one thing I can say. Fidelity and abstinence is not only required by God, it has become necessary if you want to survive. Frivolous sex today can literally kill you. Frivolous sex is spreading this disease like wildfire. Take it from someone who is dying. Take it from someone who is living through its destruction. Is it really worth it? Is it worth losing everything? The distain I have is for the power that has been given to sex. I have to rule over the desire to have sex. I refuse to allow it the power to rule over me. It has taken all it is going to receive. Sex has taken a lot. But it has not taken my relationship with Christ and the power to overcome every obstacle. I truly can do all things through Christ who strengthens me.

Let my loss be your gain. Gain a new perspective, and if it's not too late, choose to Live. And to my fellow survivors, don't beat yourself up for another moment. I have beaten myself up enough for the entire planet. And even more than me, Jesus has already been beaten, spit on, stabbed, jailed, lied on, whipped with all manner of weapons, tortured, mocked, laughed at, teased, talked about, hung on a cross, then died, took on all the sins of the world so that every sin of yours and mine can be forgiven, and in all his Glory, He rose. He was the perfect sacrifice, which mended the relationship between God and Man.

The good news for you and I is that, he got up on the third day. The sting of death no longer has the victory in your life. Don't beat yourself up another moment. Your Lord, Your Savior has already taken the ultimate beating. God truly has a purpose for your life, and as you have seen, all things truly do work together for the good for those who Love the Lord and are the called according to His purpose.

I have a new expression in life. If life gets you down, look for the ups. There truly is an up in every situation. I have lived for 22 years and counting with this disease. Getting the treatment that you need will give you a chance to live. I did not think I would live to see my children grow up, let alone graduate. But most importantly: In Christ I have found peace like you would not believe existed. God has placed all these agencies and resources to be a blessing in your life. Don't be ashamed. Take advantage of these resources. Why hide in your homes and not treat yourself with the necessary medications because you don't want anyone to find out? If they don't love you just as you are, they don't matter. If no one loves you, know that God loves you. And in the end, trust me-- He is the only one that matters. Live your life to the fullest, and serve God with all your heart, mind, and soul.

Be careful about taking advice about having a relationship with God from someone who doesn't have a relationship with God. The clue is they will tell you, you're supposed to be a Christian. If they know so much about what a Christian is supposed to do then why aren't they doing it? You have to study the word before you can tell someone what it says. And if you study the first thing you would have learned is that you don't beat someone up side their head with the word of God. If you're seeking Godly advice from someone who hasn't attended church, Sunday school, bible study or prayer meeting since their mother made them go to church, they might not be the person to get advice from. I could only guess that if we search deep into this individual we will probably find a person who is angry with the church. They're angry with someone who has hurt them. In their distorted view they believe that you think you are better than them. You do not think this way but their anger has them looking at the situation through a distorted perception. This is their problem, not yours. They will have to get help. If you are interested in having a relationship with God, seek him for yourself. You read the word. You study to show yourself approved unto God. Not unto man, but unto God. You study so you can rightly divide the word of truth.

You can't change the past. And there's no need to. The past belongs to the past. You belong to the future. And here's your promise for your future:

"Therefore if any man be in Christ, he is a new creature: old things are passed away; behold, all things are become new." (II Corinthians 5:17 kjv)

He will give you the strength to do all that He has for you to do. And when His will is done, He has promised you mansions and streets paved in gold.

"In my Father's house are many mansions: if it were not so, I would have told you. I go to prepare a place for you." (John 14:2 kjv) "The twelve gates were twelve pearls, each gate made of a single pearl.

The great street of the city was of pure gold, like transparent glass." (Revelation 21:21 kjv)

Don't let any devil in hell judge you nor convince you that your life means nothing. Don't let anyone make you ashamed of your past. Trust me, they don't want you in their closet. And they certainly don't want you in their past. Accept Him as your Lord and Savior, and you will enter in.

(I Corinthians 6: 9-11 kjv) "Know ye not that the unrighteous shall not inherit the kingdom of God? Be not deceived: neither fornicators, nor idolaters, nor adulterers, nor effeminate, nor abusers of themselves with mankind, nor thieves, nor covetous, nor drunkards, nor revilers, nor extortionist, shall inherit the kingdom of God. And such were some of you; but ye are washed, but ye are sanctified, but ye are justified in the name of the Lord Jesus, and by the Spirit of our God."

Who am I? Here is the description that God has given to me of who I am. Feel free to adopt this as your own. For God has given each of us this exact description.

"I have been washed in the blood of the lamb. I have been washed whiter than snow. I will not be

defiled. I will not allow any and everything to enter this temple. I am His, He is mine. I am satisfied in Jesus. There is nothing you can offer to turn me into a dog that goes back to lick up his vomit. I am an over comer. I am more than a conquer. I am a royal priesthood, a holy nation. Promise resides in me. I will not be deterred. Love watches me, keeps me and never forsakes me. I am a joint heir and the power to move mountains is mine. I walk in peace, I rely on his patience. His praise will continually be in my mouth; 'for I will praise thee; for I am fearfully and wonderfully made: marvelous are thy works; and that my soul knoweth right well.'" (Psalm 139:14 kjv)

I've learned a lot of lessons throughout this entire experience. I don't know what the future may hold. I pray I have grown. I pray I have helped another move from their place of loneliness and sadness.

Something happened to me that made me look at my shattered life in an entirely different manner. I had the perfect bowl. It was a quart-sized clear glass bowl, with measurement lines on each side, a pour spout and a plastic lid. It was perfect for mixing and storage. When mixing, the measurements were already on the side, so you could easily measure your contents. When pouring, the spout allowed for easy pouring, and the lid allowed for easy storage. The clear glass allowed you to easily see what was contained.

When I literally had to flee my house in Delaware I lost most of the contents when my husband broke up the furniture and trashed the house. I longed for the little things. When I returned to my home after it was destroyed I was joyful to find my favorite bowl. When my apartment was flooded, we lost probably two thirds of the contents contained in our apartment, but I grabbed that bowl.

I took it with me to the hotel where we were staying. I thought I left the bowl when I left the hotel. I called them to explain that my bowl was in their cabinet and to please go back and retrieve it. They said they checked all the cabinets and there was no bowl. I was so sad that I lost something so small but something I cherished, nonetheless.

I was complaining to everyone. One morning I reached high into the cabinet to get a plate not paying attention. When I lifted up the plate the bowl fell and shattered onto the floor. This thing didn't just break into large pieces, but it literally shattered into hundreds of little pieces. The glass covered the entire kitchen floor. Some of the pieces went onto the carpeted section of the floor.

I grabbed the broom and began to sweep. I realized I was longing after this bowl. I was sweeping with a gentleness and longing that I should not have over this bowl. At that moment I began to tell myself, just like this bowl cannot be put back together, your old life as it was can no longer be put back together.

God has promises over here waiting for me, but when am I going to let go of the shattered pieces? There is no mending what has been broken. What you long after is no longer there. Your place of rest is over here. Can you leave that broken shattered place and move to a higher place in Me?

I began to see the bowl for what it was. I had lost so much. I needed to hold on to something. Anything tangible that showed I didn't lose it all. Can I keep something? No. What you long after no longer exists.

My daughter came into the kitchen when she heard the glass break. I told her don't come in here without your shoes. I just broke my favorite bowl. I then realized that my instinct was to protect my children from the shattered pieces of my life. We don't want them to get cut; we don't want our hurts to befall them. Sometimes we hold on to the shattered pieces so long, it begins to cut so deep that it reaches them.

Over there is promise, over there is hope, over

there is healing, over there is forgiveness. Don't look back; there is nothing there for you. Come on up to this place that I have prepared just for you to start over. But I am holding on to a bowl full of old stuff.

You can start over my friends. You can buy an unused brand new bowl. My dear friends Deacon and Deaconess Phillips brought me a new bowl. I told this story in one of my sermons and they remembered. Move on from that shattered place. If it takes finding new friends and buying new stuff, then do what's necessary. The past belongs to the past. You my dear friends belong to a bright new future with all new stuff and hopefully a new bowl.

Chapter 18

<u>There Will Be Pain and Joy</u>

I do not want to end this book with the perception that everything is going to be perfect. I do not want to leave you believing that everyone in your life is going to fall in line once you tell them these stories. I am scared a lot. I pray when I am scared, but sometimes the fear does not go away. I tell myself, *"For God hath not given us the spirit of fear; but of power, and of love, and of a sound mind." (II Timothy 1:7 kjv)* But, the fear is still there. I want to know that I'll get a chance to experience so much with my children. But, I don't know if I will get that chance. I know that faith is the substance of things hoped for the evidence of things not seen. But that did not change the fact that I couldn't sleep last night. When that happens, don't feel as if something is wrong with you. You are human. You have feelings. I have faith. I believe my faith is sometimes tested. So I have to encourage myself in the Lord. I have to tell myself, "I know I am having doubts right now Lord, but yet I will trust you." I started writing today at 4:00 a.m. This was after praying since 1:00 a.m. and never being able to fall asleep. Don't think I have forgotten the promises in God's word. Those promises are confirmed to me in sermons, songs and studying his word. I will be the first to tell you Evangelist Darlene is not perfect. But she is human.

So many times I have to place myself away in a place of solitude, with just me and God. I talk to him just like he is my friend. So many people say they don't know how to pray. Prayer is just communicating with God. I tell him every fear and every concern. I ask for forgiveness, over and over again. I ask for blessings for all my friends and family. Sometimes I am relieved. Sometimes I am not. During restless nights like this I wonder how we are going to fix the car. How are we going to get the tuition? Time and time again, God has made a way out of no way. But there have been times when we just couldn't get things done. I have been struggling since I was hospitalized in 2004. God has kept my family all our lives. I have a wonderful friend who once told a lady at a flea market, who was trying to sell me some items, "She doesn't have any money, Jesus is keeping her." My first thought was, what makes you think I want this lady to know that I don't have any money. But the more I thought about it, I was in agreement. Jesus is keeping me. He is keeping me and my children. I joke with her and say I am a kept woman. Well I truly am a kept woman. I am being kept by an almighty God. It's not because of anything I have done; it's only because of His grace and mercy.

There are people who will judge you because of this disease. There are people who will shun you because of this disease. There are people who will not want to touch you. They have not educated themselves to find out that they can't catch this disease by treating you with simple love and kindness. But for the grace of God, it could be them or one of their family members. And with all these single couples having unprotected sex, it's just a matter of time before someone's number is up.

I know that people do not treat victims of this disease like they do other chronic illnesses; however, I wish they would be objective enough to recognize some of the similarities. There are other diseases that ravage the body from the inside out. They weaken the immune system and break down all of the patient's defenses. At some point, the patient begins to waste away. When this happens, people unite to surround the patient with love and kindness. We show care and concern. We hug them and touch the patient to comfort him. We know we cannot catch this illness. We have compassion and sadness. We search for ways we can help to lessen the load. We fix dinner. We clean the home. We help care for the children. We keep asking the patient, "Is there anything I can do to help you?" This is exactly the type of care and concern we should show for any patient in need. Patients should be overwhelmed with help.

I can only pray for the day when HIV/AIDS patients will be overwhelmed with help. Fear that people can contract this disease will be replaced with education. Armed with the knowledge of how we can and cannot contract this disease, our desire to help will replace our fear.

Some HIV/AIDS patients have a wonderful network of family and friends for support. They are overwhelmed with support. Yet there are those who live alone. They have no friends. They need help and assistance. We need to hasten the day when family and friends won't fear HIV/AIDS.

When I am bombarded with help, I want to be able to say to my family and friends, "There is nothing you can do for me today, but I have a friend that could use your help. My friend's body is being ravaged from the inside out. He is weak and can no longer care for himself. He now has full blown AIDS, and I am afraid he will die alone. If I could get to him I would. Don't worry you cannot catch the disease by just helping. Can you go in my place? Can you bring him some food? Please help my friend. He doesn't have any food. No one can go shopping for him until the 1st of the month. He could also really use a listening ear. He really needs your help. Please don't let my friend die alone."

I don't want to suggest for one moment that we shouldn't show every chronically ill patient all the love, care, and compassion that they need. I want us all to rush to their aid and provide all the support we can. There are many who are in a position to help. All who are willing with the capacity to give, we ask for your love and support.

Everyone is not going to fall in line and hurry to help. But my prayer for you, the reader, is that you will find a true friend or that you will become a true friend.

Some may feel that people suffering with HIV/AIDS deserve what is happening to them because of how they have lived. It's easy to forget that no one is perfect. We all deserve something for the things we have done. I may not have done the same things you have done, but we have done something. But instead of getting what we deserved, we received God's Grace. We received God's Mercy. We received God's unmerited favor. We should hope that others will also receive the same.

Being in this position, when I am all by myself I often say, "If I could turn back the hands of time..." I see so many points in my life where I would have made different choices. I had so many chances at accepting the loving advances of different mates. But then I think I would not have the same beautiful children. I would not be able to share and help others suffering from my place of experience. I would not be whom God has called me to be. Our ways are not his ways. Oh, it doesn't stop us from asking the question, why me? I have learned the long and hard way that it's me, because I can handle it. You have been placed here to help those who cannot handle it. If you had not gone through every hurt, pain, struggle, embarrassment, rejection, betrayal, longing, addiction, depression and sadness, most of the people you help would not be able to relate to you.

In all things give thanks. I am thankful that I can

be a blessing to someone else. The power of life and death is in the tongue. I want to speak life into every individual I have the pleasure of coming in contact with. Speak God's life giving love he has for all mankind. We have enough people speaking hurtful things in our lives. Some may speak things that destroy our self-esteem and self-worth. You are not by yourself. I still feel rejection today. Everyone is not so quick to give you a hug. It's okay. Focus on true friends who don't mind giving you a hug. Everyone is not willing to shake your hand. If truth be told, I am the one who should be afraid of shaking hands. I am the one with a weakened immune system. You'll catch a cold for a week. I told you about the bout of coughing and flu-like symptoms I had that lasted a year. I am sure I came in contact with someone and caught something. As I am ending this book I have just gone through a bout of pneumonia. A month later I was hospitalized with an infection. I caught this from someone I came in contact with. I am not going to stop showing others compassion. I have placed my health in God's hands.

    Be educated about this disease. Get tested for this disease. This disease is spreading because there are some who do not know their status. We can stop the spread of this disease. I and others have suffered and many have died. This is a burden you do not want to take on. Learn from our mistakes. Learn from our suffering. I ask you to Live.

I leave you with this. There will be pain and joy. I can't promise you how long it will last. In the word it tells us that *"weeping may endure for a night, but joy cometh in the morning." (Psalm 30:5 kjv)* My night sometimes feels like it has lasted the entire 22 years. Joy came one morning, unexpected and welcomed. I don't know how long your night may last, but weep as long as you need to. See every burden being released through those tears. There will be pain, sorrow and regret. I feel them all. But no one can tell you how long your night will last. When your night is over, Joy will come in the morning. Embrace your joy.

About the Author

Darlene King is an HIV survivor from Philadelphia. She grew up in a loving environment where God was always first and caring for others was a natural second. The love and support she continually receives from her family strengthens and guides her life's work daily. The pain of all she has experienced has been poured onto the pages of this book.

Darlene is a born again Christian. She was trained and licensed as an Evangelist in Philadelphia. She has also graduated from the Evangelism Institute. Darlene currently serves on the Ministerial Staff. She has served as Worship Leader, Youth Director, Director of Vacation Bible School, Youth New Members Instructor, Discipleship Training Instructor, Evangelism Institute Instructor, Sunday School Teacher and Administrative Assistant to the Senior Pastor. She served as Director of Responsive Strategies to Violence Prevention, a program she developed for youth in Southwest Philadelphia. Darlene has facilitated many workshops over the years for youth and adults, and has spoken at many churches and colleges on HIV/AIDS awareness and shared her personal experience.

She volunteers with Action Aids of Philadelphia on the Speaker's Bureau program as well as various volunteer assignments as needed. Darlene has committed her life to serving others living with HIV and AIDS by being a voice for those who may not have a voice because they have been scared into silence. She is an advocate for those who have been shunned, a friend for those who may be lonely, a confidant for a down bent shoulder, and a hand to lift those up who have been shut out.

God has blessed her to live to experience and see things she could have never imagined. Through her trails she has gained a greater understanding of (Psalm 37:25 kjv) *"I have been young, and now am old; yet have I not seen the righteous forsaken, nor his seed begging bread."* To God she gives ALL the Glory.

You may contact Darlene King via e-mail at:
Darleneking13@hotmail.com

or on Twitter:
@darleneking13

www.ingramcontent.com/pod-product-compliance
Lightning Source LLC
Chambersburg PA
CBHW022104160426
43198CB00008B/339